G158

W9-BTB-047

Reflexology

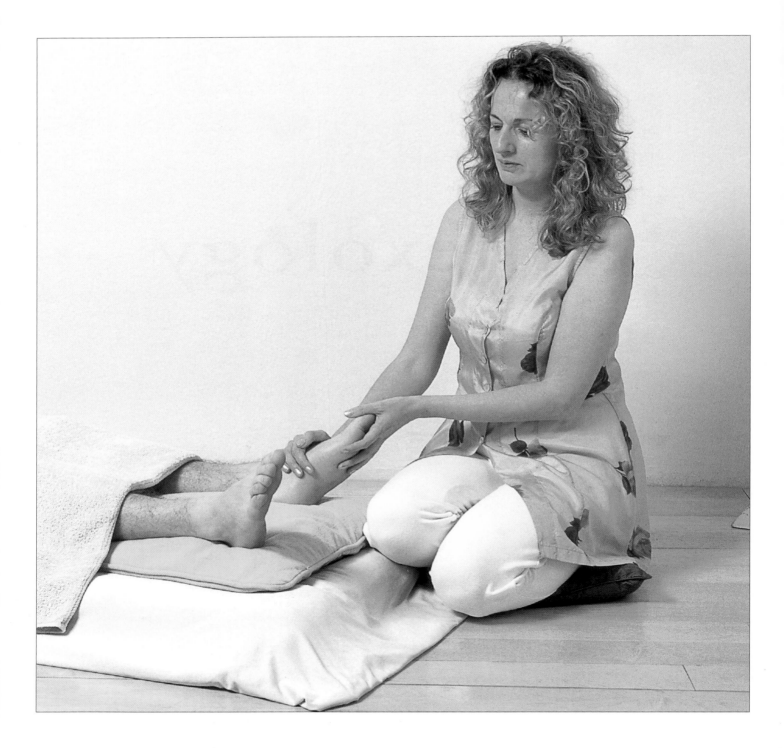

Reflexology

A practical introduction

Denise Whichello Brown

Eagle
Editions

A QUANTUM BOOK

Published by Eagle Editions Ltd
11 Heathfield
Royston
Hertfordshire SG8 5BW

Copyright ©MCMXCIX
Quantum Publishing

This edition printed 2000

ISBN 1-86160-377-0

QUMAIRX

This book is produced by
Quantum Publishing
6 Blundell Street
London N7 9BH

Printed in Singapore by
Star Standard Industries Pte Ltd

contents

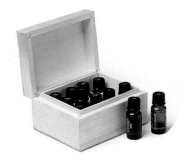

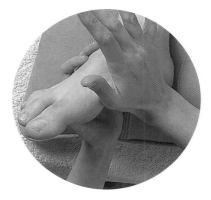

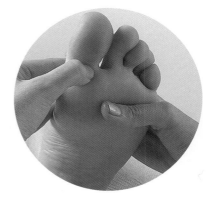

introduction to
Reflexology

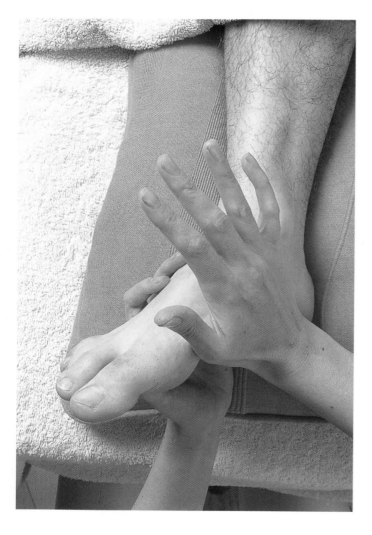

Pressure applied to areas on the feet can influence corresponding regions of the body. This simple movement encourages the spine to relax.

Reflexology is a simple, non-invasive, harmless and natural way to optimum health. It is easy to perform, and no special equipment is required in order to practice it. All you need are your hands and a willing partner. Firm pressure is applied through the thumbs and fingers to reflex points which are located on all parts of the feet. By applying pressure on these points, all the organs, glands and structures of the body can be stimulated and encouraged to heal.

This book will enable the complete beginner to soothe away the stresses and strains of everyday life and promote well-being. It will also allow you to alleviate a whole host of common conditions such as headaches, backache, digestive problems, menstrual problems, arthritis, coughs and colds, insomnia and much more. It is important to realise, however, that reflexology should not be used instead of orthodox medical treatment – if problems persist then medical advice should be sought. Reflexology must also never be used to diagnose illness. Diagnosis is the prerogative of the doctor.

Reflexology has enormous physiological and psychological benefits on all the systems of the body.

THE BENEFITS OF REFLEXOLOGY

1.   Reflexology induces relaxation

Stress is a part of our everyday life, and if we do not manage stress properly then the body's defences break down, making us more susceptible to illness. It is generally conceded that 75% to 80% of ailments are attributed to stress and reflexology is capable of inducing a state of deep relaxation and tranquillity. The alpha state of relaxation is generated during a treatment which leads to a level of consciousness at which healing can take place. During a reflexology session most people will fall asleep and awake refreshed and restored with a wonderful sense of well-being and inner harmony.

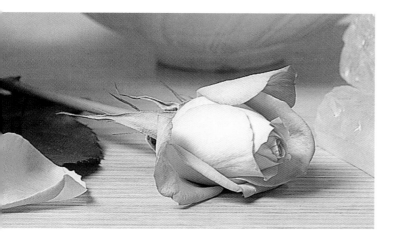

Calming accessories can aid relaxation.

2.   Reflexology is preventative health care

Reflexology boosts the immune system and thus prevents illnesses and diseases from occurring. As the reflex zones on the feet are treated, the natural healing forces within the body are released and mobilised, restoring the body to harmony. Since the time of Hippocrates, health has been defined as a balanced state and disease as an unbalanced state or dis-ease. Instead of passively waiting for the harmony to fall into disorder, which allows health problems to develop, reflexology aims to achieve this homeostasis. Patients who receive regular reflexology treatments report that they are far less susceptible to catching colds and flu even though everyone around them may be coughing and sneezing. Reflexology has effectively strengthened their immunological defences and thus enhanced their health.

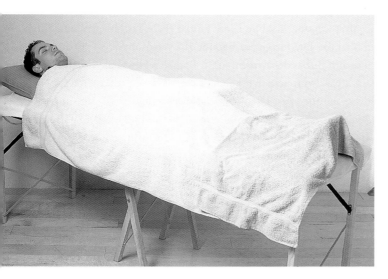

A reflexology treatment is so relaxing that the patient often falls asleep.

3.   Reflexology improves the circulation

It is vital for blood to flow freely throughout the body as it carries essential oxygen and nutrients to the cells. Circulation can become sluggish and the blood flow can be restricted and impeded. Reflexology can improve the blood flow to every part of the body.

4.   Reflexology detoxifies the body

The lymphatic system and the systems of elimination such as the colon, kidneys and skin are responsible for the detoxification of the body. If they are not functioning properly then toxins will build up. These waste deposits can be palpated by sensitive fingers on the reflex zones of the feet like small grains of sugar and can be broken down by reflexology massage and eliminated.

5   Reflexology revitalises energy

Reflexology regenerates and opens up energy pathways, revitalising the body and supplying it with renewed and invigorating energy. We are all very much aware of when our 'batteries' are low, and many individuals feel tired and lethargic all the time. It is vital that we recharge our batteries with reflexology as often as we are able.

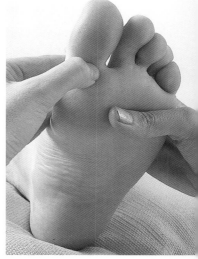

6   Reflexology improves mental function

Toxins can be identified as small grains, and broken down during a reflexology treatment.

Reflexology calms the mind and relieves it of all unnecessary 'clutter'. Thus mental alertness is restored, thoughts can be clarified and new ideas can be stimulated.

7   Reflexology stimulates emotional release

Reflexology can adjust emotional imbalances in the body. During treatments, unresolved emotional problems are encouraged to rise to the surface and can then be dealt with. Many physical ailments stem from an emotional source. Negative states of mind will block the free flow of the life force and cause disease. As the old, unwanted emotions are released, changes in attitude and personality often take place and balanced health is restored.

origins and principles of Reflexology

Reflexology is an ancient therapeutic treatment for activating the innate healing powers of the body. Ancient techniques of pressure have been practised for thousands of years by many different cultures. It is widely thought, although never proven, that reflexology has its origins in China over 5,000 years ago. However, the first evidence depicting the practice of reflexology comes from Egypt. In Saqqara, in the tomb of Ankmahor, an Egyptian physician, an ancient painting which dates back to around 2330 BC depicts treatments of the hands and feet actually taking place. The hieroglyphics are as follows:

"Do not let it be painful." (patient)
"I shall act so you praise me." (practitioner)

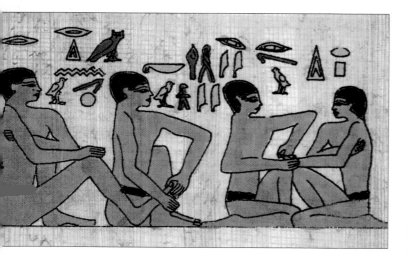

Illustration from Ankmahor's tomb in Saqqara, Egypt. Dated around 2330 BC.

Our modern concepts of reflexology originated with the zone therapy of the American physician Dr. William Fitzgerald (1872-1942). Born in Connecticut, he graduated from the University of Vermont in 1895 and practiced at Boston City Hospital, the Central London Ear Nose and Throat (E.N.T.) Hospital and also in Vienna. Dr. Fitzgerald became the head physician in the ear, nose and throat department at St. Francis's Hospital, Connecticut and it was from here that he made the medical profession aware of his 'zone therapy'. Dr. Fitzgerald discovered that if pressure was applied to specific areas or points on the body, an anaesthetic effect could be induced. Not only could pain be relieved but also the conditions producing the pain.

In 1917 Dr. Fitzgerald, together with his colleague Dr.Edwin Bowers, published a book entitled 'Zone Therapy, Relieving Pain at Home', and devised a dramatic demonstration for convincing sceptics of the theory's validity. First they applied pressure to a volunteer's hand, then stuck a pin into the anaesthetised area of the person's face – with no apparent pain.

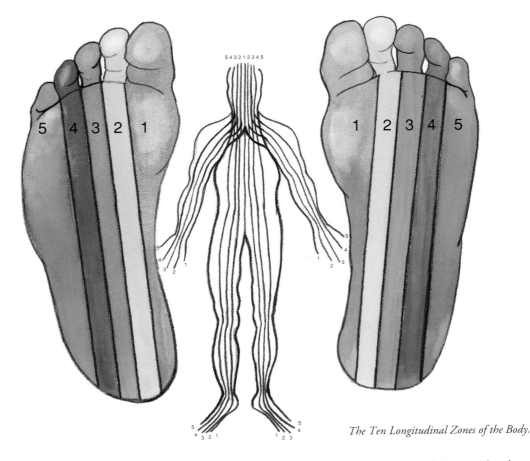

The Ten Longitudinal Zones of the Body.

In this book, Fitzgerald divided the body into ten longitudinal zones of equal width running the length of the body from the tips of the toes to the head and out to the fingertips and vice versa. He claimed that if a line is drawn through the centre of the body there are five zones to the right of this mid-line and five zones to the left of it. Zone one runs from the big toe, up the leg and centre of the body to the head and then down to the thumb. Zone two runs from the second toe, up to the head and down to the index finger. Zone three extends from the third toe, up to the head, down to the third finger and so on. All organs and parts of the body lie along one or more of these zones. Stimulating any part of a zone in the foot by applying direct pressure affects the entire zone throughout the body.

Dr. Fitzgerald's theories began to spread across America. Although many in the medical profession were sceptical about his work, Dr. Joseph Shelby-Riley, a chiropractor, was a true believer. Fitzgerald taught zone therapy to Shelby-Riley and his wife Elizabeth who were both keen practitioners. Dr.Shelby-Riley wrote several books including 'Zone Therapy Simplified', (1919). He is renowned for introducing Eunice Ingham, a physiotherapist, to zone therapy.

Eunice Ingham (1879-1974) is considered to be the founder and mother of modern reflexology. It was through her work that foot reflexology was born in the early 1930s. In 1938 she published 'Stories the Feet Can Tell', followed by the sequel 'Stories the Feet Have Told'. These classic texts are still used by reflexologists today.

She mapped out the entire body on the feet which she viewed as being a mirror or a mini-map of the body. When Eunice retired in the 1970s after dedicating her life to reflexology, her work was continued by her nephew Dwight Byers.

Reflexology was introduced into Britain in the 1960s by Doreen Bayley (1900 - 1979) who had trained with Eunice Ingham.

Apart from the longitudinal zones, the feet can also be divided into transverse or horizontal sections. Transverse zones were first described by the German reflexologist, Hanne Marquart, who also trained with Eunice Ingham. The four transverse lines are as follows:

A. The shoulder girdle line located just below the base of the toes.
B. The diaphragm line located just below the ball of the foot.
C. The waist line in the middle of the foot in the centre of the arch of the foot.
D. The pelvic line just above the heel.

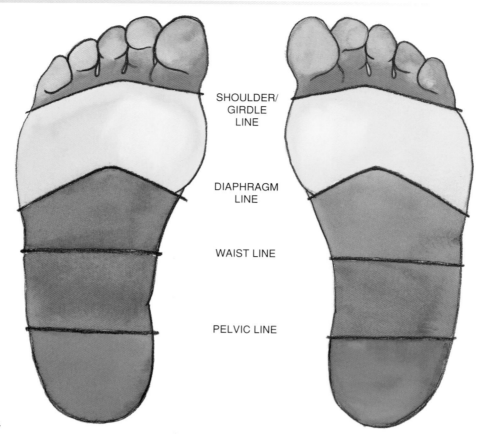

SHOULDER/
GIRDLE
LINE

DIAPHRAGM
LINE

WAIST LINE

PELVIC LINE

The Four Transverse Zones.

These imaginary lines help us to map out the body on the feet. All the organs and structures of the head and neck lie above the first transverse zone – the shoulder girdle line.

All organs above the diaphragm on the body will be represented above the diaphragm line on the foot.

All organs below the diaphragm are found below the diaphragm line on the foot.

The feet precisely mirror the body. The right foot corresponds to the right hand side of the body, while the left foot reflects the left hand side. Paired organs such as the lungs, kidneys or ovaries are found one in each foot. Single organs such as the liver or spleen are found either in the right or the left foot according to where they are located in the body.

The spine, which is in the centre of the body, is found in both feet along the inside (medial aspect) of the foot. Outer parts of the body such as the shoulders, knees and hips are found on the outside (lateral aspect) of the foot.

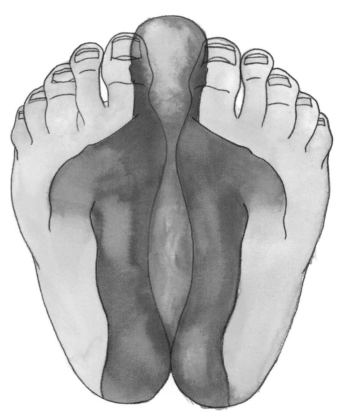

The Feet Mirror the Body.

Getting started

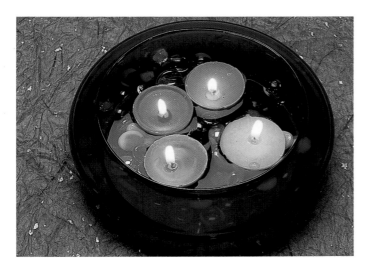

Candles can enhance the ambient atmosphere needed for reflexology.

CREATING THE RIGHT AMBIENCE

Reflexology does not require any complicated or expensive equipment. All you need are your hands, your intuition and the desire to help others. Although reflexology can be performed almost anywhere it is well-worth creating the right environment to allow the recipient to derive maximum benefit from a treatment.

The surroundings should be as peaceful as possible. As the aim of your treatment is to induce relaxation, the noise of telephones, children or traffic will not help create a healing atmosphere. Take the telephone off the hook and make sure that your family know that you are carrying out a treatment. Some people will enjoy listening to relaxation music in the background during their reflexology. Others will prefer silence to help them relax. It is entirely up to individual preference.

SETTING OUT YOUR ROOM

The room should be very warm and inviting. Although only shoes and socks are removed, some loss of body heat is inevitable as the treatment progresses. Warmth will encourage feelings of security and relaxation. Lighting should be soft and subdued. Bright lights should be dimmed or even switched off and replaced with candles. Tinted bulbs can also provide the perfect setting. You may wish to burn some essential oils or some incense prior to your treatment or have a vase of fresh flowers in the room to enhance the environment.

Small clay burners for diffusing essential oils are readily available and reasonably priced. Put a few teaspoons of water into the loose bowl on the top and sprinkle a few drops of your chosen essential oil into it. Light the night light and allow the wonderful aromas to diffuse into the atmosphere. Suitable essential oils for creating an atmosphere of relaxation include lavender, clary sage, geranium, jasmine, neroli, ylang-ylang or rose.

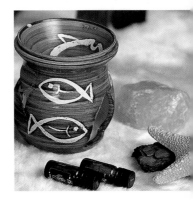

A few drops of soothing aromatic oil in a burner provide an added effect.

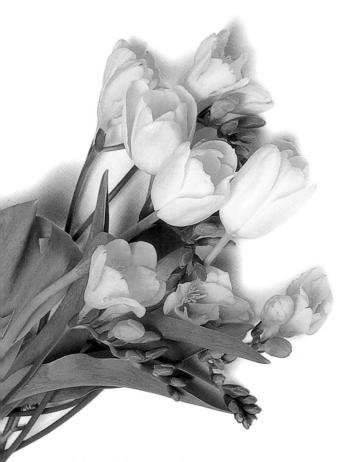

Fresh flowers help create a relaxing environment.

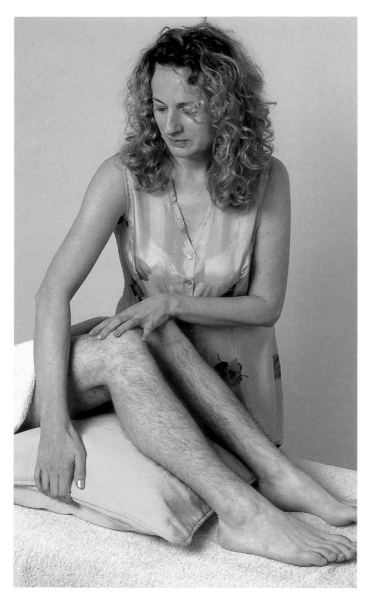

Place a pillow under the receiver's knees for added comfort.

It is important to sit with a correct posture in order to perform reflexology effectively.

POSITIONS FOR WORKING

A professional reflexologist will use a massage couch but it is not essential to buy one. You may decide to invest in one later on but for home use, a bed is all that you require. The receiver should lie down with his/her feet at the foot of the bed. Pillows should be placed under the head to support the neck and to allow you to observe any facial expressions. You may also wish to place a pillow under the receiver's knees to take any pressure off the lower back. A pillow or cushion placed under the foot that you are working on may be useful for your own comfort. It is important that you are just as relaxed as the receiver.

Position yourself on a swivel chair or a stool within easy reach of the receiver's feet in a relaxed upright manner. Your legs and knees should be slightly apart, your feet on the ground and your shoulders should be down and relaxed. If there is any tension in your body then the receiver will almost certainly be aware of it. Tense hands cannot move smoothly, and they will be unable to feel any abnormal reflex areas in the feet.

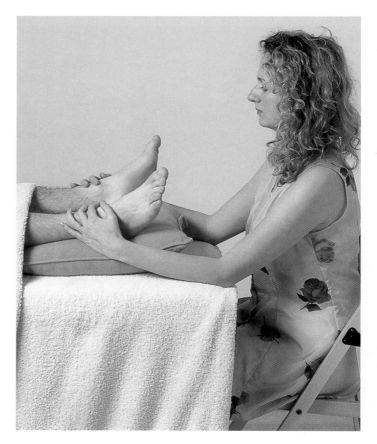

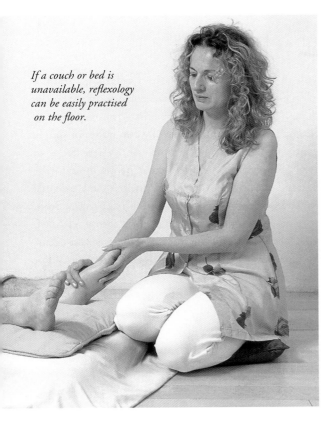

If a couch or bed is unavailable, reflexology can be easily practised on the floor.

You may prefer to work on the floor using a well-padded surface. Place a thick duvet or two or three blankets on the floor. Either kneel or sit cross-legged and rest the receiver's foot on your lap or on a pillow. You will still need pillows or cushions under the receiver's head and the knees.

Some people like to work with the receiver sitting on a chair but this will not suit everyone. It is not as comfortable for either the giver or the receiver. It also seems to encourage conversation and it is important to keep talking to a minimum for best results. Relaxation is essential to allow both of your energies to flow freely throughout the treatment.

A light blanket or towel should be used to cover up the receiver even though the clothes are not removed. As the treatment progresses there will be some loss of body heat.

Any restrictive clothing such as ties and belts should be removed to allow the energies to flow freely. You should also remove any jewellery from your hands to avoid scratching. Ensure that your fingernails are closely clipped to avoid any discomfort. Always remember to wash your hands both before and after a treatment.

Ensure hands are clean and nails are clipped before beginning a treatment. Remove jewellery.

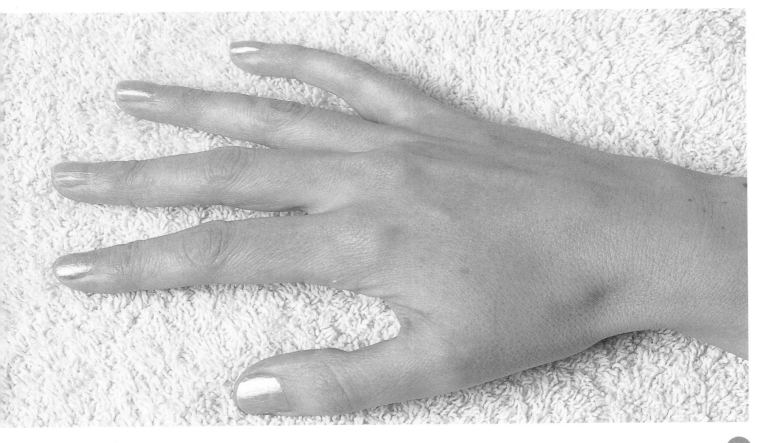

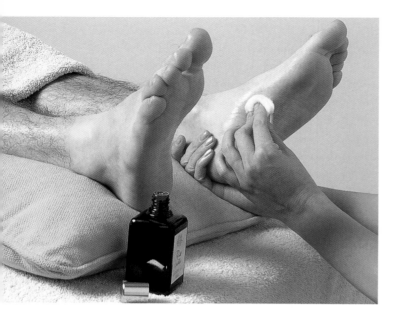

Rosewater is ideal for cleansing the feet.

REFRESHING THE FEET

You may wish to cleanse the feet prior to a reflexology session. Sweaty, unpleasant smelling feet can cause embarrassment to the receiver and are not pleasant to work on either. You may want to soak the feet for a few minutes in a bowl of warm water, or simply wipe feet gently with moist cotton wool. Add a few drops of essential oil of lavender, tea tree, lemon or peppermint to the water to relax and cleanse feet. If you do not have any essential oils you may add a sprig of fresh lavender or peppermint from your garden or squeeze some fresh lemon juice into your bowl. Rosewater is excellent for cleansing the feet. However you decide to refresh the feet always dry them thoroughly. Avoid using oils or creams during your treatment. Too much lubricant will make it difficult for you to hold the foot properly and will cause your walking thumb or finger to slip. A barrier will also be created, decreasing your sensitivity and making it difficult for you to detect any abnormalities. Some people use talcum powder on the feet, but this can be messy, and may block up the pores.

Essential oils should never be applied undiluted to the skin. To make up a massage blend just three drops of essential oil are added to two teaspoons of cold-pressed, unrefined, additive-free carrier oil such as sweet almond or apricot kernel. You may prefer to add your essential oils to a pure organic skin cream in the same dilution. To a 30gm amber coloured glass jar add up to 9 drops of essential oil to create an excellent foot cream.

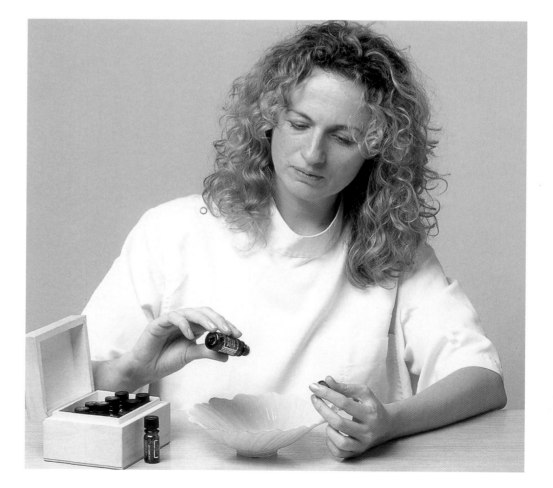

Oils can be mixed to create an individual massage blend to be used at the end of the treatment.

REACTIONS FROM REFLEXOLOGY

Both during and after a reflexology treatment, physical and psychological changes may occur. All responses should be seen as positive and highly desirable as reactions show that the body's self healing mechanism is being activated. The body is trying to expel unwanted toxins. Reactions have been divided into those which may occur during a treatment and those which may appear between treatments.

Possible reactions during a treatment

- Changes in expression
- Visible contraction of the muscles e.g. shoulders
- A feeling of deep relaxation and the desire to sleep
- A warm glow as energy blockages are released
- Feelings of euphoria
- Sensations of the body expanding and spreading as it relaxes
- Shooting sensations as blockages release
- Running nose if the head zones are being treated and are blocked
- Twitching or tingling
- Warmth in the area of the body being worked on

Possible reactions between treatments

- A state of deep relaxation
- An alteration in sleep patterns eventually leading to deep sleep
- More frequent and noticeable dreams
- Emotional changes with a greater awareness of feelings
- Increased skin activity – pimples, rashes, increased perspiration. Eventually skin tone and texture improves
- Increase in urination
- Cloudy or unpleasant smelling urine
- Bowels move more frequently
- Increase in bulk and volume of the stools
- Nasal discharges
- Coughing and secretions from the bronchi
- Colds
- Sneezing
- Watery eyes
- Sore throat
- Fever
- Vaginal discharges
- Toothache
- A need to drink more water to flush away the toxins
- Previous illnesses which have been suppressed may flare up temporarily and then disappear.

IMPORTANT – these reactions NEVER occur simultaneously.
After a treatment one or two reactions MAY occur.

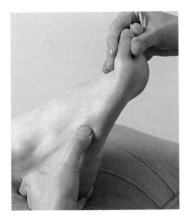

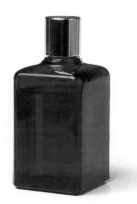

Contraindications to Reflexology

NEVER USE REFLEXOLOGY IN THESE CIRCUMSTANCES:

- Immediately after surgery until the doctor has pronounced complete recovery
- When the receiver is suffering from a fever – the body is already fighting off toxins and a reflexology treatment would release more toxins into the system
- If the receiver has an infectious skin conditions such as scabies, as you do not want to spread the condition or infect yourself. NB: Conditions such as eczema and psoriasis are NOT infectious and should improve with treatment.
- If the receiver suffers from thrombosis – reflexology could move a clot
- During pregnancy where there is an element of risk especially during the first 12-14 weeks or if the pregnancy is complicated

Be careful of:

- Corns and calluses – use gently pressure if they are painful
- The pancreas reflexes when treating a diabetic
- Pressure when treating a diabetic. Use less pressure, as the skin can be thinner, bruises easily and diabetics may heal more slowly
- The heart area if there are cardiac problems or if the receiver has a pacemaker
- Over treating any one particular area
- After a heavy meal – wait a couple of hours before treatment

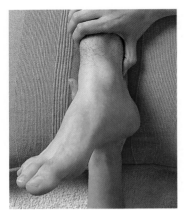

Never:

- Diagnose or promise to cure a condition
- Apply strong pressure. A treatment should NEVER be painful
- Press directly over a cut, bruise, recent scar, painful area or severe varicose vein

basic reflexology Techniques

I n this chapter you are going to learn the basic techniques which you will be using in your reflexology routine. Please ensure that your nails are trimmed before you start so that they do not scratch or dig into the receiver's foot. Reflexology should NEVER be painful. Your pressure should be firm yet not uncomfortable. If the receiver flinches or tries to withdraw his or her feet then you are pressing too hard. Every individual's feet will be different – some are much more sensitive than others. As you work, use your intuition and watch the facial expressions of the person receiving treatment. Adjust your pressure accordingly.

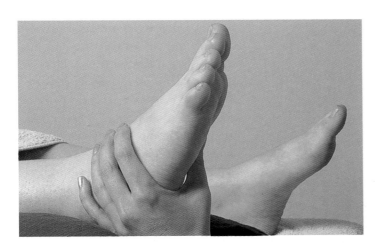

HOLDING TECHNIQUE

To be a good reflexologist it is important to hold the foot correctly so that the reflex zones can be easily reached, accurately pinpointed and stimulated. You need to develop good teamwork between your hands as you will always be holding and working the foot with your two hands. One hand is used to support and hold whilst the other hand will work the reflexes.

To work on the right foot place the heel of your left hand against the outer aspect of the foot. Wrap the fingers of your left hand lightly over the front of the toes and the thumb under the back of the toes.

This position allows you to support and control the movement of the foot very effectively. The foot can be pushed backwards away from you brought towards you or even twisted slightly.

Practice this holding technique on the left foot too. This time your right hand will act as the holding hand leaving your left hand free to work on the reflexes.

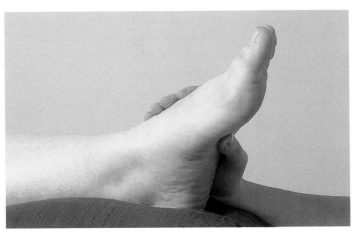

> ### REMEMBER
> Do not grip the foot too tightly

THUMB/CATERPILLAR WALKING TECHNIQUE

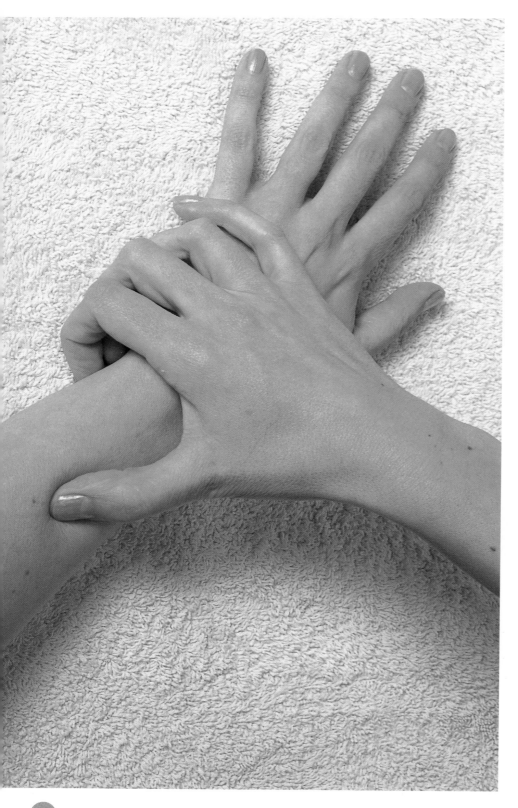

This movement is performed with the outer edge of the thumb.

To find this point place your hand palm downwards onto a table and notice the tip of the thumb that touches the surface of the table – this outside tip is to be the working area of your thumb.

Strength in reflexology is made possible by the appropriate use of leverage, and leverage is achieved by the use of the four fingers in opposition to the thumb. First of all practice the caterpillar walking on the palm of your hand or on your forearm.

To walk the thumb bend ONLY the first joint of the thumb slightly and then unbend the joint slightly. Only allow the thumb to take very SMALL steps as it walks along the hand/forearm. The walking movement is always performed forwards never backwards nor sideways. You should aim to maintain a constant, steady and even pressure. An on-off-on-off pressure should not be felt at each bend of the thumb. Do not worry if your thumbs start to ache or feel sore at first. With practice your thumbs will increase in tolerance and build up strength. Do not be discouraged – be patient and keep trying. As the thumb is walking, the four fingers should be moulded to the contours of the hand/forearm. The four fingers should be kept together comfortably to ensure maximum leverage. If they are spread out then some of the leverage will be lost.

Then practice thumb walking up each of the five zones along the entire length of the foot. Ensure that you are holding the foot correctly with your supporting hand wrapped around the toes. Work from the base of the heel in zone five up towards the base of the little toe – see sequence 1–3.

Now work from the base of the heel in zone four up towards toe four and repeat this thumb walking up each of the other zones. Then walk up each of the five zones on the other foot – see sequence 4–6.

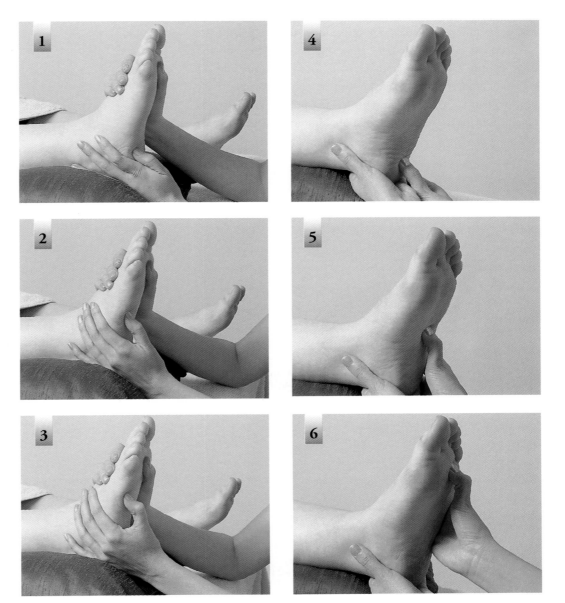

REMEMBER

- Ensure that you are holding the foot properly
- Use the outer edge of the thumb
- Do not dig your nail into the skin
- Bend only the first joint of the thumb slightly

- Employ a constant, steady pressure NOT on-off-on-off pressure
- The thumb always moves FORWARDS, never backwards or sideways

FINGER WALKING

The finger walking technique is basically the same as the thumb walking technique. The first joint of the index finger is used.

Excellent places to practice your finger walking are on the back of your hand or on your forearm. Use the corner edge of your index finger as you walk forwards taking the smallest bites possible while exerting a constant, steady pressure. Leverage is obtained by the use of the thumb in opposition to the fingers.

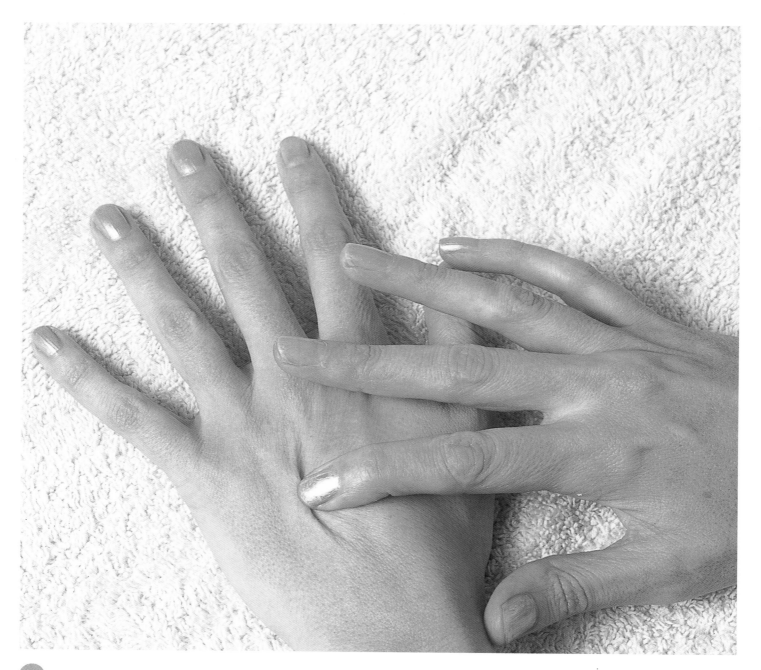

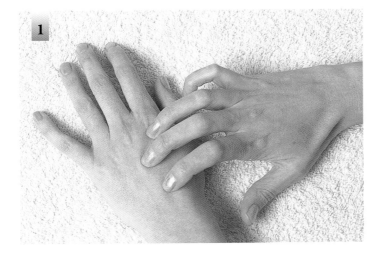

Once you have mastered finger walking with the index finger, try using your other fingers. (1) Any finger may perform this technique.

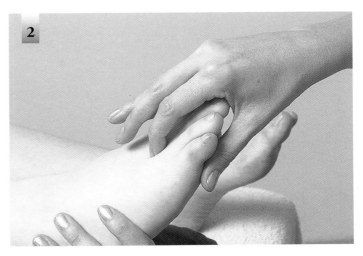

Now try the technique on the receiver's foot. Usually only one finger is used at any one time (2).

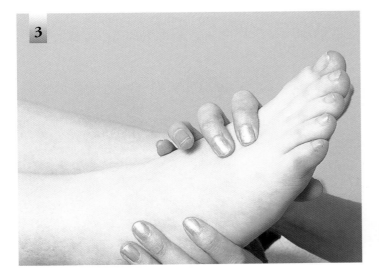

However, two or more fingers may sometimes be used, for example when working across the top of the foot (3).

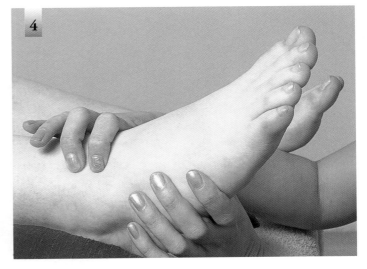

Finger walking is the most appropriate technique when working on bony and sensitive areas such as the top of the foot and around the ankle (4).

REMEMBER

- Take only very small steps to cover the area
- Do not dig in your nails or press too hard

- Always move your index finger **forwards**, not backwards or sideways

HOOK IN AND BACK-UP/PINPOINTING TECHNIQUE

This technique is used to apply pressure to specific points, and requires great accuracy. Certain points on the feet are either too small or too deep for the walking techniques to be used effectively. However, this very precise technique should never be employed when covering a large area. It is ideal for contacting the tiny reflex points such as the pituitary gland which is found on the big toe.

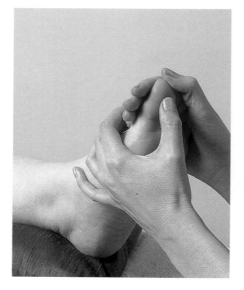

Once again the outside edge of your thumb will be your contact point.

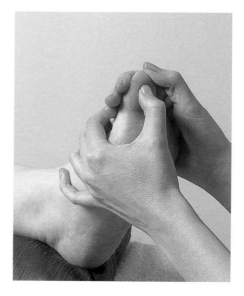

Place the thumb of your working hand onto your chosen reflex point. Apply pressure with your thumb to this point. (In this case the pituitary gland).

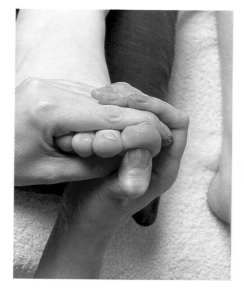

Now pull back across the point with the thumb. Push in, then back up. You may repeat this technique several times.

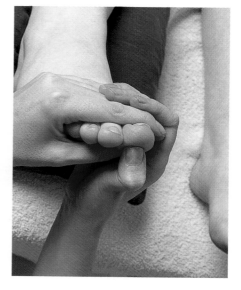

This technique has been likened to a bee inserting a sting. A bee lands on a spot and backs the stinger into your flesh. Your thumb lands on a small point and hooks in and backs up.

REMEMBER

- Never use the very tip of your thumb otherwise your nail will dig in
- Use the flat pad part of the outside edge of your thumb

PRESSURE CIRCLES ON A POINT

This technique is particularly recommended for working on tender reflexes or sensitive areas on the foot.

Hold the foot comfortably with one hand and place the flat pad part of the thumb of the other hand onto the tender area. Here the solar plexus area is illustrated. Press slowly into the area and circle your thumb gently over the area several times. After a few pressure circles any tenderness should have diminished.

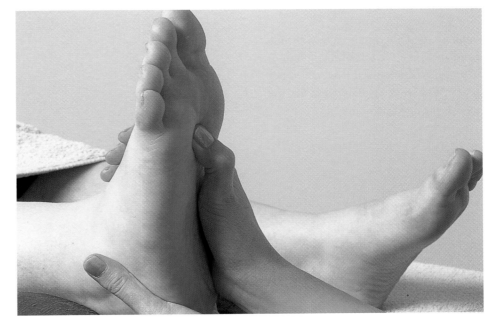

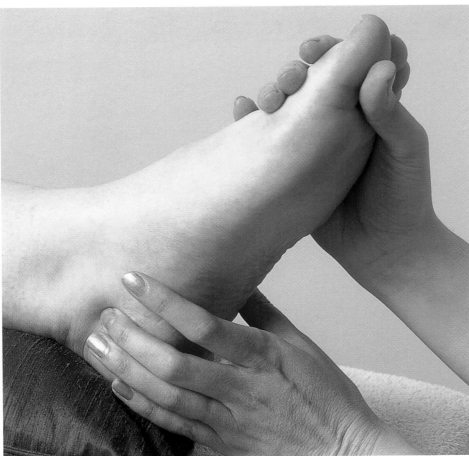

The thumb is always used for this technique apart from the uterus/prostate and ovary/testicle points where the index or the third finger is used. Here the uterus area is illustrated.

REMEMBER
- Do not dig in with your fingernails
- If the tenderness does not diminish, leave the area and return to it later

ROTATION ON A POINT

This technique may also be used on any tender reflexes.

Support the foot comfortably with one hand and place the pad of the thumb of your other hand onto the relevant reflex point. With your holding hand, flex the foot slowly into the thumb.

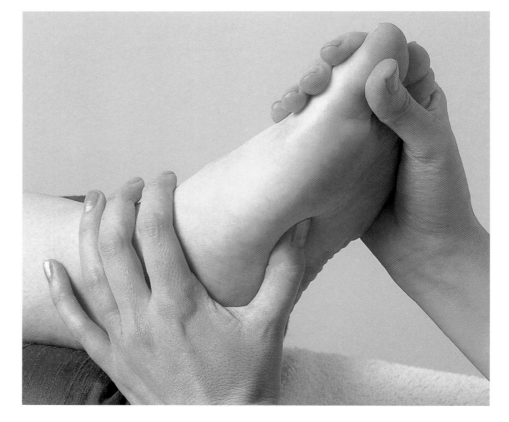

Rotate the foot in a circular motion around the thumb. In this illustration the technique is performed on the kidney reflex.

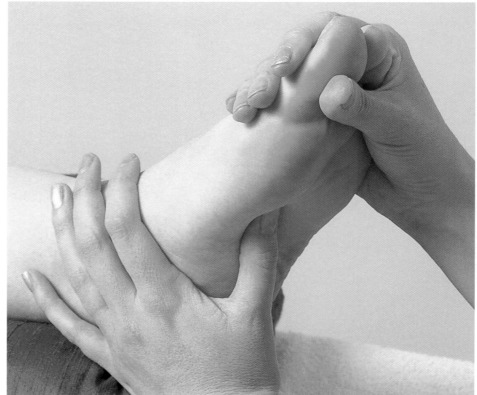

REMEMBER
- Rotate the foot slowly with your holding hand for maximum relaxation
- Ensure that you are not digging in with your thumbnail
- Do not allow your thumb to slip off the reflex point

reflexology relaxation
Techniques

Relaxation techniques are always used prior to a reflexology treatment. They are designed to put the receiver at ease and to help to establish a relationship of trust. Someone having their feet worked on for the first time is bound to feel a little nervous and often worries that the treatment will feel ticklish. These techniques will help to dispel any initial nervousness. They will also loosen any muscular tension in the feet and make them soft, supple and easy to work on.

Use these techniques in any order, and repeat some of them throughout your reflexology treatment. It is not necessary to master all of them so choose your favourites. As your confidence grows it is quite acceptable to create your own.

Use a few relaxation techniques at the end of a complete treatment as a 'dessert' to enable the receiver to gain maximum benefit and pleasure.

TUNING INTO THE FEET

To begin the relaxation sequence, hold both feet. Take a few deep breaths allowing all the tension to flow out of your body. You should be able to and feel the receiver completely relax.

As you tune into the person you are treating, imagine the healing energy flowing freely through your hands and body.

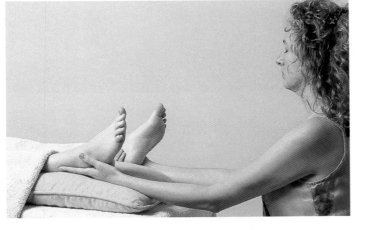

REMEMBER
- Use no oils or creams for your preliminary relaxation sequence (although they may be used at the end of the treatment)
- Make sure that you remove rings, bracelets and watches before you work
- Check that fingernails are short and even

EFFLEURAGE/STROKING

Using both hands, stroke the whole foot firmly covering both the top, the sides and the sole of the foot.

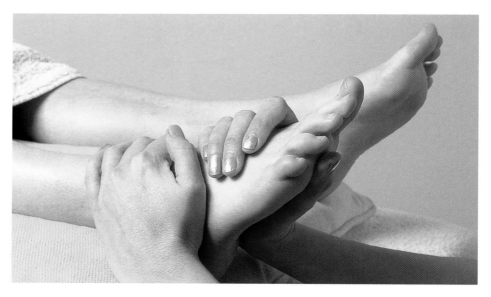

Work up from the toes, gliding around the ankle bones and back again.

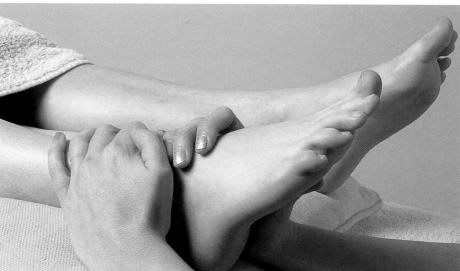

Repeat this movement several times. Stroking relaxes, increases blood flow and helps to disperse any excess fluid especially around the ankles.

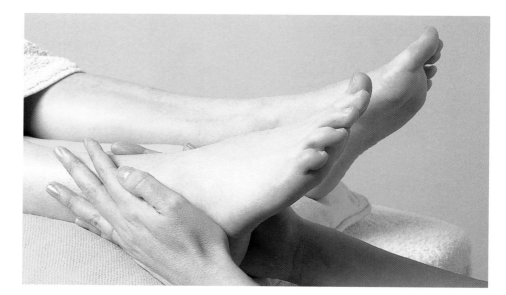

METATARSAL KNEADING

If working on the left foot, hold the top of the left foot with your right hand just below the base of the toes. Your hand should 'wrap' around the foot, with your thumb on the sole of the foot and fingers on the top of the foot. Make a fist with the left hand and place it on the fleshy area on the ball of the foot.

Work from the ball of the foot to the heel using a gentle circular motion.

This technique helps to soften the tissues on the sole of the foot.

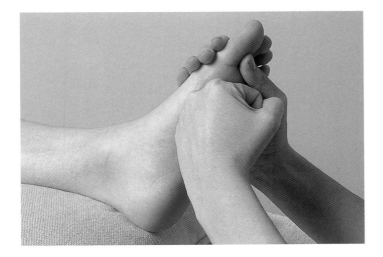
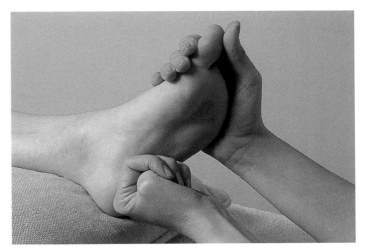

ALTERNATE THUMB ROTATIONS

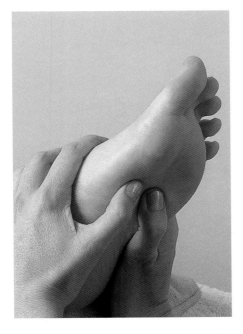
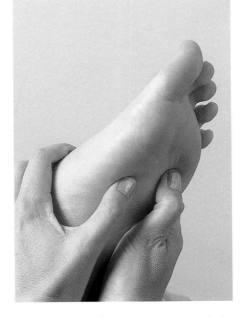
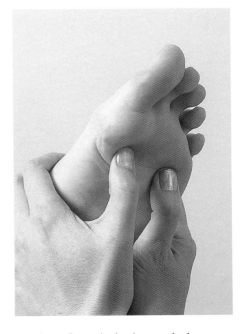

Grasp one foot with both hands so that your thumbs are on the bottom of the sole of the foot and your fingers are on the top.

Rotate one thumb at a time using small circular movements – alternate right thumb clockwise, left thumb anti-clockwise.

Work up from the heel towards the toes.

ZIG-ZAG/SPREADING THE FOOT

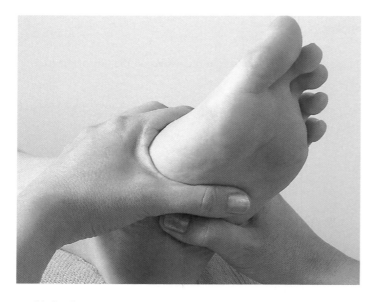

Hold the foot with both hands so that the balls of the thumbs are placed flat against the sole and the fingers are flat on top – one hand will be slightly higher than the other.

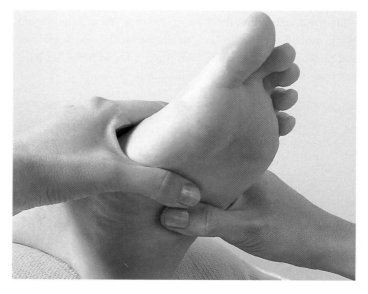

Pull the thumbs away and past each other towards the edges of the foot and then allow them to slide back towards each other.

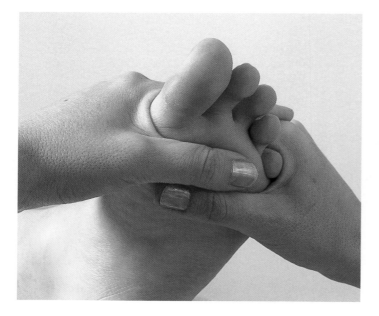

Work the thumbs in this zig-zag movement from the base of the toes to the base of the heels and back again.

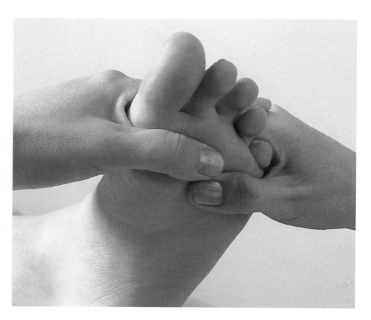

Feel that you are opening out the foot.

FANNING THE SPINE (SPINAL STROKING)

Cup the heel of one foot so that it is resting in the palm of your hand. This holding technique is first illustrated on the left foot to show hand position clearly.

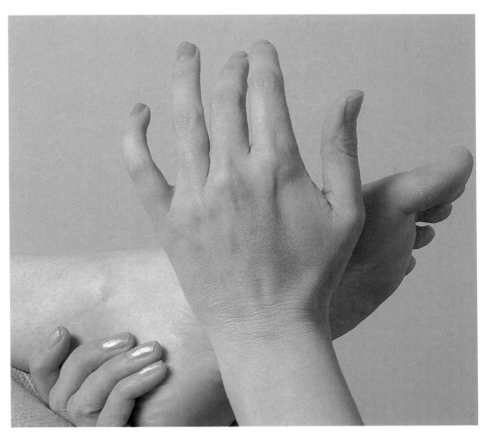

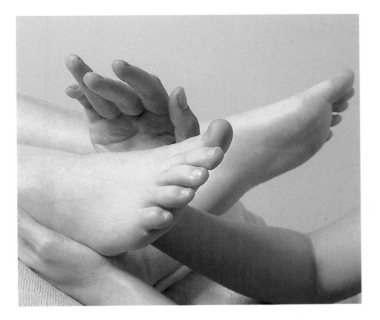

With the heel of the other hand stroke firmly down the inside (medial aspect) of the foot working from the big toe towards the heel. This movement is illustrated on the right foot.

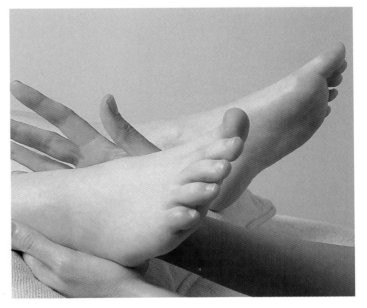

As the inside edge of the foot corresponds to the spine, this technique will encourage the spine to relax and is excellent for neck and back pain sufferers.

SPINAL TWIST/PUSH AND PULL

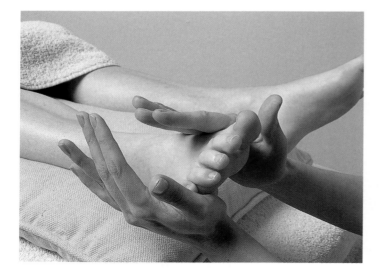 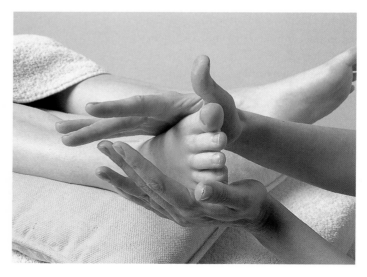

Place one hand on the inside of the foot and your other hand on the outside of the foot. Using the heels of the hands pull the outside of the foot towards you with one hand as you push the inside of the foot away from you, and vice versa.

Work along the edges of the foot from the heel to the toes and back down again. Perform these movements slowly to further relax and improve mobility in the spine.

Twisting the bottom of the foot loosens the lower back and working either side of the ball of the foot loosens the upper back and alleviates stiffness in the shoulders.

TOE LOOSENING

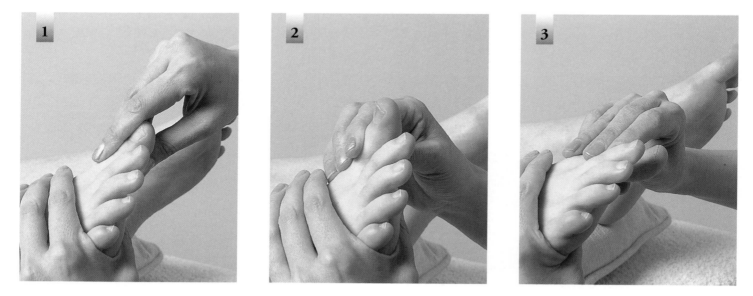

Support the foot gently with one hand, thumb on the sole of the foot, fingers wrapped around the top of the foot. Using your thumb and index finger close to the base of each joint, gently stretch each toe and then rotate each toe both clockwise and anti-clockwise (sequence 1–3) This technique will increase the flexibility of the toes and will also loosen the muscles around the neck and shoulders.

ANKLE ROTATIONS

Support the heel in one hand, thumb on the outside of the ankle, fingers on the inside.

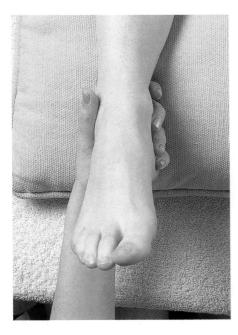

Grasp the top of the foot in your other hand and slowly and gently rotate the ankle several times in one direction (1) and then in the other direction (2). This movement helps relaxation, and increases mobility in the lower back and pelvis.

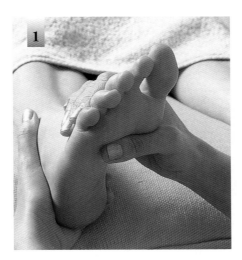

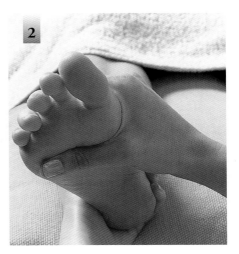

FOOT ROCKING

Place the palms of your hands one either side of the foot. Move them alternately and rapidly from side to side so that the foot vibrates.

This movement stimulates circulation and relaxes the muscles in the foot, ankle and calf.

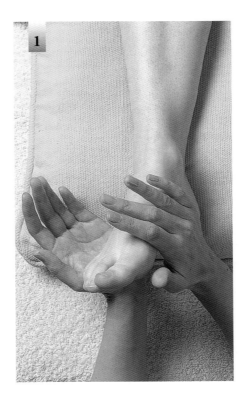

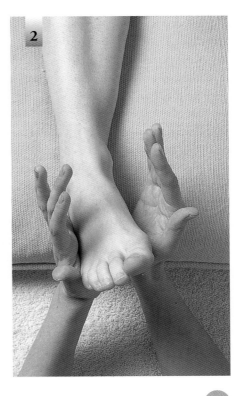

LOWER BACK RELEASE

Grasp under the heels of both feet.

Lean backwards, and slowly and gently pull the feet towards you. Release the stretch just as slowly.

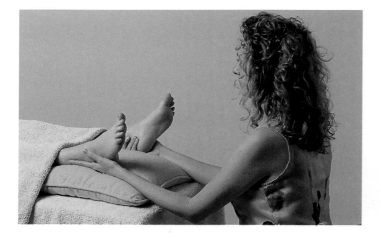

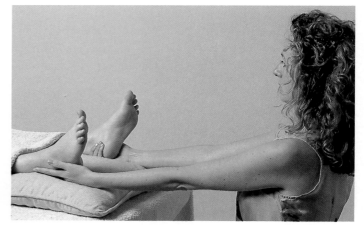

SOLAR PLEXUS/DIAPHRAGM RELEASE

The solar plexus is the main area which stores our stress and tension. Applying pressure to this area encourages a state of relaxation and also helps the breathing to deepen and slow down. This is the ultimate in relaxation techniques. It should always be used to complete a treatment. The solar plexus release may be performed on one or both feet.

To locate the solar plexus, place one hand over the top of the upper part of the foot and squeeze gently. A hollow will appear on the sole of the foot at the diaphragm line this is the solar plexus (1).

Release the foot, remembering where this point is. Now find the solar plexus on the other foot.

Take the left foot in your right hand and the right foot in your left hand, fingers on top, thumbs on the bottom. Place your thumbs onto the solar plexus reflex. Press the solar plexus reflex very gently and slowly (2). Hold for a few seconds. Release your pressure gradually but do not lose contact with the feet. Do this several times.

You can synchronise this technique with the receiver's breathing. Ask them to take a deep breath and, as they do, press into the solar plexus. As they slowly breathe out you should release your pressure on the points.

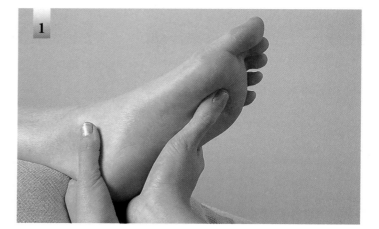

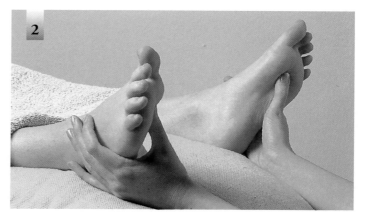

beginning a reflexology
Treatment

INTRODUCTION

Now that you have familiarised yourself with the basic techniques and have mastered some of the reflexology relaxation techniques you are ready to work on the reflex points.

Remember that you should never diagnose conditions – this is the prerogative of the medically qualified only. Reflexology is not a substitute for orthodox medical treatment. If the receiver has a problem which does not resolve then always seek the advice of a medically qualified doctor.

LENGTH OF TREATMENTS

The timing of treatments and the amount of pressure used varies from individual to individual depending upon their needs. A complete treatment with practice will probably take you about 45 minutes. For your initial treatment allow at least an hour. When working on a child, the younger the child the shorter the treatment. A baby would only need a five minute treatment consisting of stroking movements whereas an older child of 12 would be able to receive about 30 minutes. A treatment would also be shorter if you are working on elderly or very sick people. Reflexology is suitable for all ages and it is rare to find someone who will not benefit from treatment.

Do not be tempted to spend too long on a treatment. If the session is too lengthy then there is the possibility of overstimulating the body. This could cause excessive elimination resulting in diarrhoea or some other uncomfortable condition.

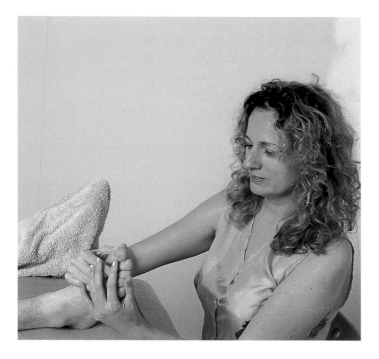

A complete treatment should be around 45 minutes, but individual's needs may vary.

HOW MUCH PRESSURE TO USE

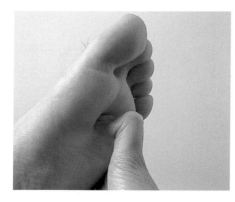

Applying excessive pressure can cause pain or discomfort.

It is important to work very gently during the first treatment session in order to see how the person reacts. The amount of pressure required will vary from one individual to another. If your partner feels as if he/she is being tickled then more pressure is needed. If the feet are jerked backwards away from you, then obviously you need to reduce the intensity of your treatment. Once you have established the right pressure you should sustain it evenly throughout the session.

It is interesting that a person will not necessarily always require the same amount of pressure. Factors such as emotional trauma or hormonal changes could well result in the feet becoming more sensitive. If the person is highly stressed or very debilitated then again light pressure should be used. Drugs such as painkillers or any medication that de-sensitises feeling will make the feet less sensitive.

As conditions improve you will probably find that you can use firmer pressure. However this does not mean that sensitive reflexes indicate an unhealthy person and insensitive reflexes mean a healthy person. Some unhealthy people can have very insensitive reflexes, whereas some healthy people have very tender feet.

Always stroke the foot at frequent intervals throughout the treatment. This is not only very pleasant and relaxing but also will help to disperse any toxins which have been released

WHAT TO DO IF AN AREA IS PAINFUL

If you discover any tender reflexes on the feet you should only use GENTLE pressure over these areas for a short time. Treatment should NEVER be applied continuously over the same reflex point. It is far more effective (and more comfortable) to return to any painful areas at frequent intervals and to return to them at the end of the treatment. Any uncomfortable areas should eventually disappear as health and balance are restored.

NUMBER OF TREATMENTS

After the first treatment it is highly likely that an effect will be experienced. Most reactions are very pleasant but some minor irritations may be felt as the body rids itself of any toxins. Any adverse reaction should pass within 24 hours. For optimum results and especially where there are minor ailments you should try to treat the receiver once a week for approximately seven treatments. Carrying out a complete treatment more than once a week is not recommended as this could result in an area being overstimulated. After the initial sessions, depending on how much time you have, once every 2 – 4 weeks is quite adequate.

If you want to pamper the receiver with more sessions it is quite acceptable to use the relaxation techniques as often as you like.

WHAT A TREATMENT FEELS LIKE

On the whole a treatment is extremely pleasurable and very addictive. Most people will fall asleep during a treatment which is excellent for healing. However, they may experience some strange sensations. Several people report feeling needle-like sensations, while others can experience a dull ache in certain areas of the foot. Tingling sensations may also be felt as blockages are released. Overall, however, your receiver will feel incredibly relaxed yet light and revitalised by the end of the session.

Stroking feet regularly will relax the receiver, as well as dispersing toxins.

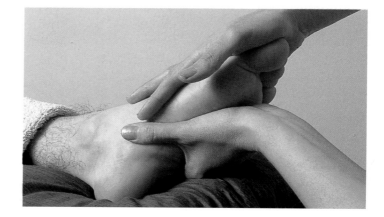

THE TREATMENT

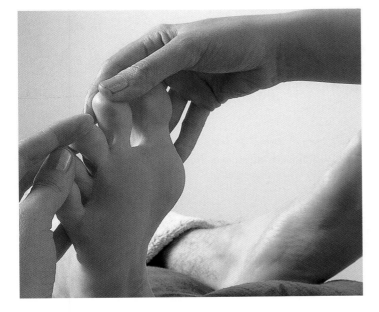

Check feet for tender areas before beginning treatment.

You are now ready to begin. Ask the receiver to lie on the bed or couch, make them warm and comfortable and if necessary cleanse the feet. Check for any cuts, bruises, corns, verrucae, ingrowing toenails etc. which could be tender or contagious. You will need to work gently on these areas or even avoid them altogether. Remember to always cover the foot you are not working on.

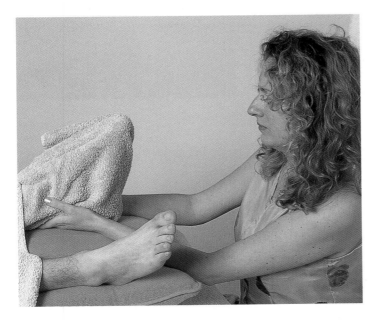

When working on one foot, always keep the other warmly wrapped.

PERSONAL PREPARATION

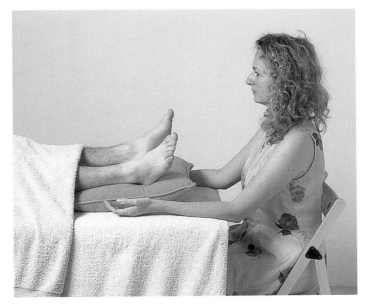

Ensure that you are calm and relaxed before beginning a treatment.

Before commencing your reflexology massage it is important to prepare not only the environment and the receiver but also yourself. You need to centre yourself, and clear your mind of all thoughts. Consciously release all tense areas of your body particularly your neck, back and shoulders. To do this take a few deep breaths and as you exhale feel the tension melting away leaving you relaxed and calm. As you breathe in draw in healing energy.

The order of the sequence can be simplified as follows:
1. Relaxation techniques
2. All toes – the head and neck area
3. Inside of the foot – the spine
4. Ball of the foot – the chest, breast, lungs, thyroid etc.
5. Arch/instep of the foot – the abdominal area containing organs such as the stomach, pancreas, intestines, kidneys etc.
6. Outside of the foot – joints such as the knee, hip, elbow etc.
7. Heel – the pelvic and leg reflexes
8. Ankles – the reproductive area and lymphatics
9. Relaxation techniques

Thus, you are going to work each foot in a logical manner from the toes down to the heels.

RELAXATION TECHNIQUES

These techniques have already been described in detail in the previous chapter. Here only the basic movement for each technique is illustrated. Remember to always tune into the feet before beginning.

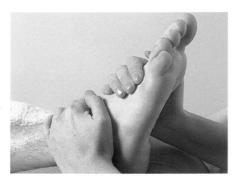

Effleurage/stroking

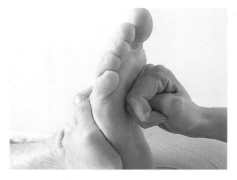

Metatarsal kneading

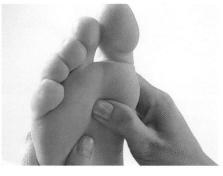

Alternate thumb rotations

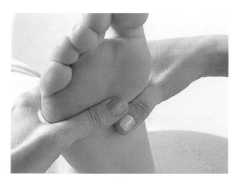

Zig-zag/spreading the foot

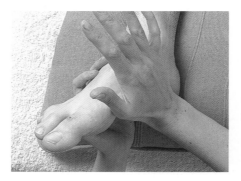

Spinal stroking

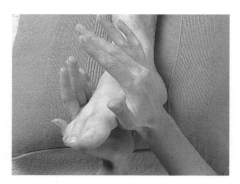

Spinal twist

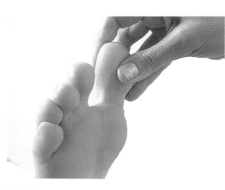

Toe loosening

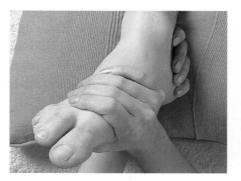

Ankle rotations

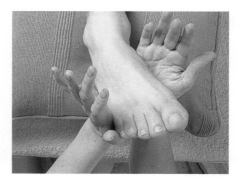

Foot rocking

TENSION RELEASE

STEP 1 DIAPHRAGM/SOLAR PLEXUS

This is the primary area for the release of tension. To locate it gently pull the toes backwards with your holding left hand to make the diaphragm line more visible. Place the fingers of the working hand on the top of the foot for leverage.

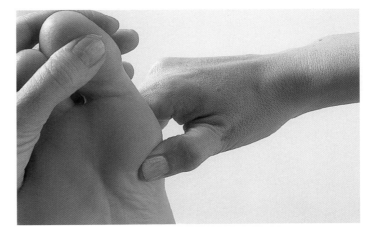

Thumb walk across the diaphragm line working from the medial aspect (inside) of the foot towards the outside.

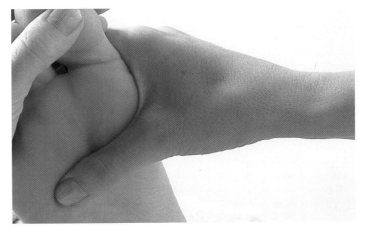

When you reach the solar plexus press gently into it as the recipient breathes in and release the pressure as the recipient breathes out. Repeat several times.

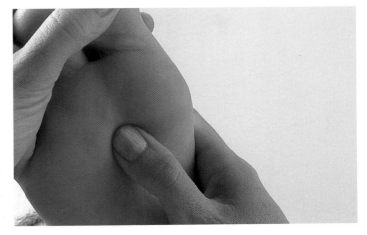

USES: relaxation and release of tension

HEAD AND NECK AREA

STEP 2 HEAD AND BRAIN AREA (BACK AND SIDES OF THE BIG TOE)

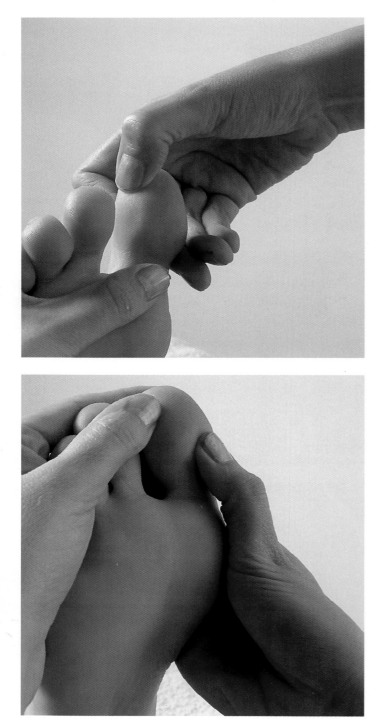

Place the heel of your left hand around the outer aspect of the foot. Wrap the fingers of your left hand over the front of the toes and your thumb under the back the toes. Using your right thumb, walk from the outer edge of the base of the big toe up the outside, over the top and down the inside of the big toe.

Now walk up the back of the big toe from the base to the tip. You will probably need to walk up the big toe three to five times to cover the entire area. If you prefer you may walk down the big toe instead of up.

USES: Working the head and brain is particularly useful for conditions such as headaches and migraine. Also for any problems affecting the brain such as defects in memory, lack of concentration or inability to think clearly.

STEP 3   PITUITARY GLAND (BIG TOE)

To find the pituitary gland reflex point, locate the widest point on each side of the big toe and imagine a line stretching across these points. The pituitary gland is found approximately at the mid-point of this line. You often have to search around to find this point. Place the fingers of your left hand over the front of the toes and your thumb under the back of the toes. With the corner of your right thumb use the hook in and back-up technique on the pituitary gland reflex.

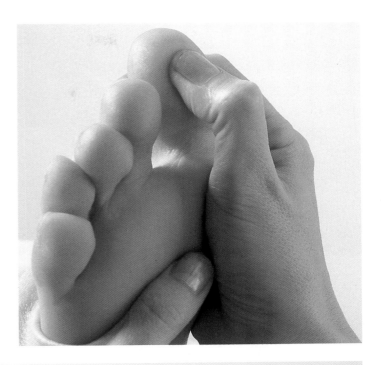

USES: All hormonal problems. (This point is often out of balance)

STEP 4   FACE (FRONT OF THE BIG TOE)

Wrap your left hand around the top of the foot, thumb underneath, fingers on top. Using your right index finger, walk down the front of the big toe from the tip of the big toe to the base. Caterpillar walk down as many times as it is necessary to cover the whole of the front of the toe.

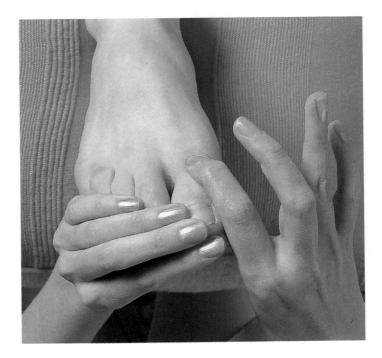

USES: Any facial problems, e.g. neuralgia, eye, nose, mouth, teeth, gum and jaw problems.

STEP 5   NECK (BASE OF THE BIG TOE)

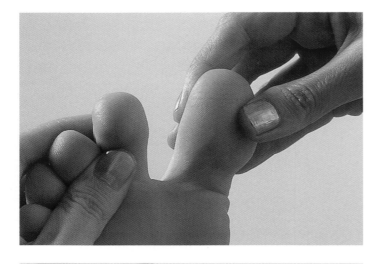

First of all of rotate the big toe. Support the foot with your left hand, hold the big toe between the thumb and index finger of your right hand and rotate it clockwise and anti-clockwise. This is equivalent to rotation of the neck. Do this movement slowly and gently. If the toe grinds or cracks or is limited in movement as you move it, this indicates a problem with the neck.

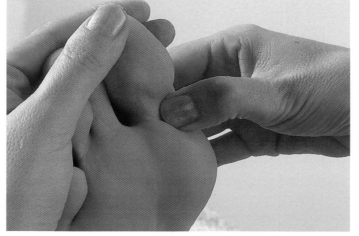

To loosen the neck further, gently grasp the big toe between the thumb and fingers of your left hand and with your right thumb walk across the back of the base of the big toe from the outside to the inside to treat the back of the neck

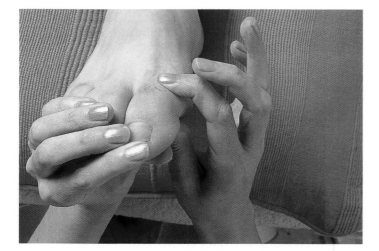

Now using your index finger walk across the front base of the big toe working from the outside to the inside.

USES: All neck disorders, problems with the throat, tonsils and vocal chords, thyroid and parathyroid.

STEP 6 SINUSES (BACK, SIDES AND TOP OF THE SMALL TOES)

To work the sinuses you are going to walk down the centre and two sides of the small toes. Support the recipient's right foot between the thumb and fingers of your left hand – thumb on the sole of the foot, fingers over the front of the toes for support and control. Starting at the top of each toe using very small steps thumb walk down to the base of each toe or even both together.

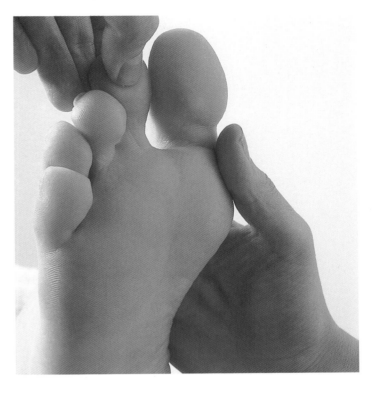

When treating the sides you may use your thumb or index finger or both together. Do this movement three times covering the centre and sides of each toe. You will probably find that working the sides of the toes is more difficult, but persevere.

This technique can also be performed by working up the back and sides of the toes, instead of down.

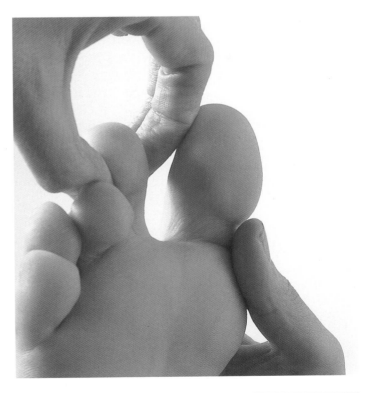

USES: sinus problems, headaches caused by sinus congestion, hay fever, catarrh and allergies.

STEP 7 TEETH (FRONT OF THE SMALL TOES)

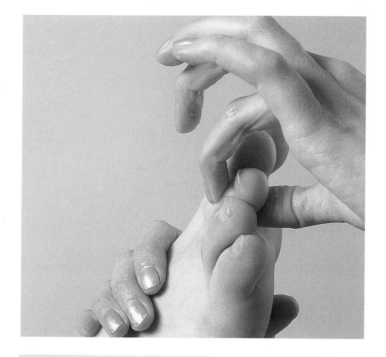

Starting at the base of the nail finger, walk down the fronts of the toes covering the centre of each toe and both sides of each toe from top to bottom.

USES: toothache, sensitive, painful or infected gums.

STEP 8 UPPER LYMPHATICS (BETWEEN THE TOES)

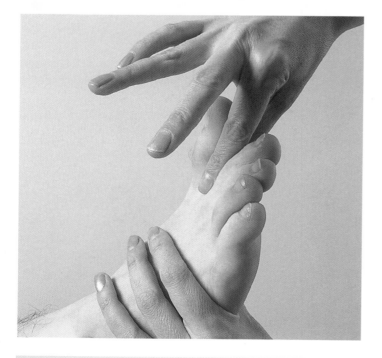

The reflex areas to the upper lymph nodes are found in the webbing between the toes. Support the foot with your left hand and with the thumb and index finger of your right hand very gently squeeze between each of the toes.

USES: to fight off and to prevent any infections.

STEP 9   SPINE (INNER EDGE OF THE FOOT)

The spinal reflexes run along the inner edge of each foot from the base of the big toes to the inner ankles. To thoroughly relax the spine, support the right foot in the palm of your left hand and stroke down the inside of the foot working from the big toe down to the heel.

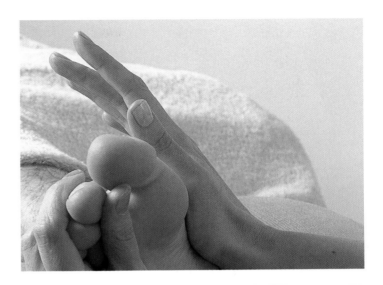

Support the foot under the heel with your holding hand and caterpillar walk down the medial aspect (inside) of the foot beginning at the base of the toenail (1). This represents the top of the spine (cervical area) and as you walk down the foot you are covering the middle of the back (thoracic area) and the low back (lumbar area) (2).

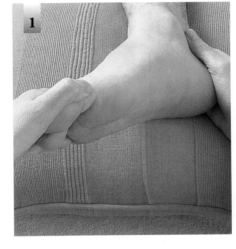
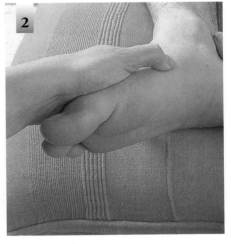

Now change hands, placing your holding hand at the top of the foot with your thumb on the back of the toes and your fingers wrapped around the front of the toes. Repeat the thumb walking working in the opposite direction from the base of the heel up to the base of the toenail.

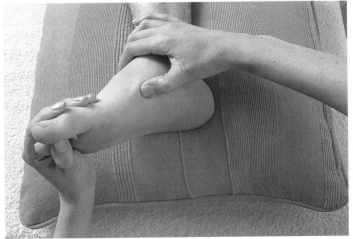

USES: All back problems, lack of mobility, arthritis, disc problems. Pain and stiffness should be greatly reduced.

STEP 10   EYES AND EARS (BASE OF THE TOES)

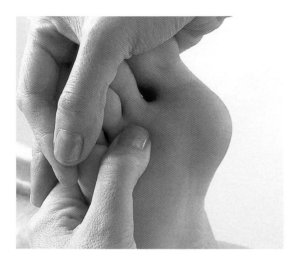

You are going to thumb walk along the ridge at the base of the toes – the shoulder girdle line. Pull the toes gently back with your holding hand to make the area easy to reach – thumb on the bottom fingers at the top. Thumb walk across the ridge moving in both directions.

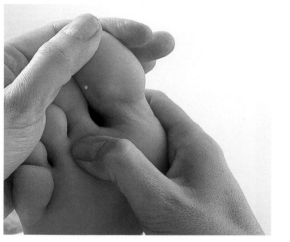

To locate the right eye more precisely, caterpillar walk across the ridge and stop between the second and third toes. Use your thumb and use the hook in and back up technique to press firmly into the eye point.

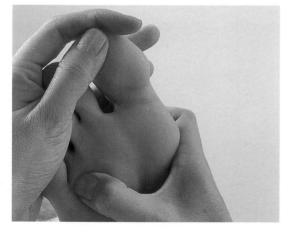

Continue to caterpillar walk and stop between the fourth and fifth toes. Press firmly into this area to treat the right ear.

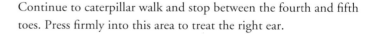

USES: sore, tired or watery eyes, glaucoma, conjunctivitis and eyesight problems.
Earache, glue ear, tinnitus, hearing problems, vertigo and dizziness.

SHOULDER GIRDLE LINE TO DIAPHRAGM LINE

STEP 11 THYROID/PARATHYROID/THYMUS

The thyroid and parathyroid reflex points are located on the ball beneath the big toe. Support the toes of the right foot back with the left hand. Place your right thumb just below the ball of the foot on the inside and thumb walk from the diaphragm line in a curved direction up to between the big toe and the second toe. Return to the diaphragm line and caterpillar walk up the foot several times until you have completely covered the area under the big toe. The thyroid is located in the centre of the pad of the ball of the foot below the big toe. As this reflex is often tender we will do pressure circles on this area.

Place the flat pad of your thumb onto the thyroid area and circle your thumb gently over the area several times. If there is any tenderness it should diminish after a few pressure circles.

The parathyroid area is found slightly to the left of the thyroid gland. Move your thumb slightly to the left and perform pressure circles on the parathyroid area.

The thymus is found to the right of the thyroid gland close to the spinal reflexes. Move your thumb to the right almost as far as the inside of the foot and once again use your thumb to circle over the thymus area.

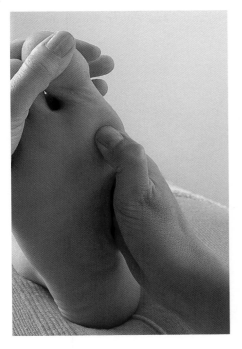
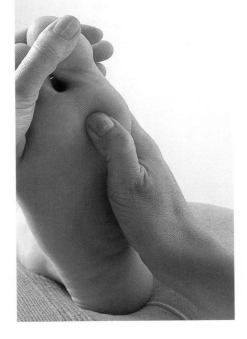
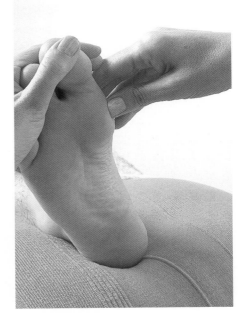

USES: thyroid problems, weight problems, nervousness, palpitations, dry skin, lethargy, menopause.
The thymus gland is important to maintain a healthy immune system

STEP 12 RIGHT LUNG/CHEST (BALL OF THE FOOT)

The lung area encompasses the entire ball of the foot from the shoulder girdle line to the diaphragm line. Pull the toes back slightly with the left holding hand with the fingers cupped over the front of the toes. Start at the base of the toes and with your right thumb caterpillar walk into vertical strips from the diaphragm line to the shoulder girdle line on the sole of the foot. Thumb walk until the whole of the area between the shoulder girdle line and the diaphragm line has been covered.

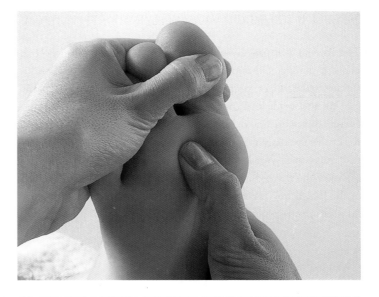

USES: coughs and colds, asthma, bronchitis, emphysema, shallow breathing, hyperventilation and panic attacks.

STEP 13 RIGHT BREAST/LUNGS/MAMMARY GLANDS (TOP OF THE FOOT)

Pull the toes forward with your left hand, thumb under the sole of the foot, fingers cupped over the top of the toes. Finger walk down the troughs on the top of the foot from the base of the toes to the diaphragm line. Cover the entire area in vertical strips. As the top of the foot is more sensitive use your index finger to do the walking. You may also use several fingers at once.

Alternatively you can support the foot by making a fist with your left hand and placing it under the toes. Finger walk in the same way as before.

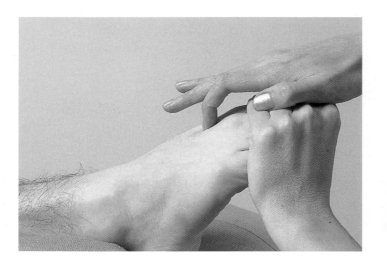

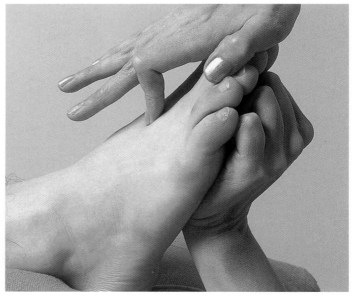

USES: respiratory problems as described in step twelve, breast problems such as tenderness due to P.M.T, harmless lumps which have been investigated

DIAPHRAM LINE TO THE WAISTLINE

STEP 14   LIVER/GALLBLADDER (RIGHT FOOT ONLY)

The liver is the largest organ in the foot and therefore has a large reflex area. Imagine a triangle extending up across the diaphragm line from the left hand side of the diaphragm line to the left hand side of the waistline and then across to the right hand side of the diaphragm line. Bend the toes away from you to open up the reflex area and caterpillar walk this whole area in diagonal strips in both directions.

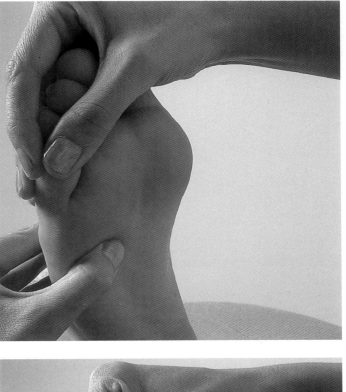

Locate the gallbladder reflex which lies in between the diaphragm line and the waistline in line with the fourth toe. The gallbladder reflex appears to vary somewhat in its location but it can feel like an indentation or a small swelling. As this is often a tender point we will use the rotation technique. Support the foot with your right hand and place the pad of your left thumb onto the gallbladder reflex. With your right holding hand flex the foot slowly into your left thumb and rotate the foot in a circular motion around the thumb.

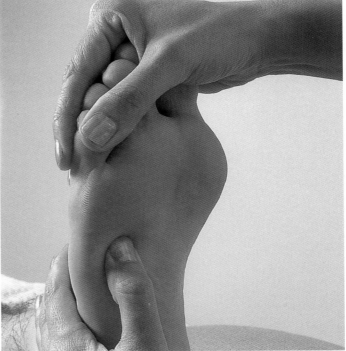

USES: digestive problems, detoxification, assists in breaking down fats, stress.

STEP 15 STOMACH/PANCREAS/DUODENUM

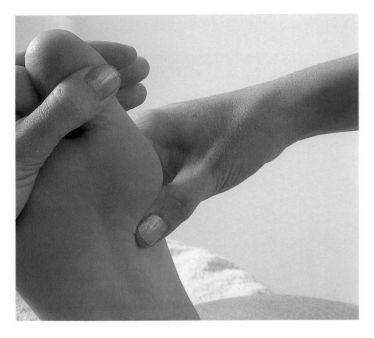

The stomach, pancreas and duodenum may be treated by working on the sole of the right foot as well as the left foot. Use your left hand to hold the foot and thumb walk just below the diaphragm line from the inside of the foot (zone one) to approximately the centre of the foot (zone three).

Repeat the caterpillar walking in horizontal rows until you reach the waistline. You may reverse the hands to work in the opposite direction if you wish.

USES: stomach problems such as indigestion, hyperacidity, ulcers and stomach cramps

STEP 16 ADRENAL GLAND

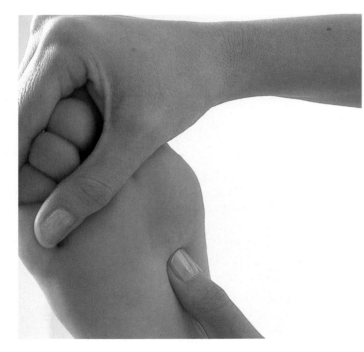

The adrenal gland is usually easily pin-pointed as it is often tender. If you pull back the toes a thick tendon will protrude running from the big toe to the heel. The adrenal reflex point is located midway between the diaphragm and the waistline on the medial side (inside) of this tendon.

With your right hand holding the right foot, fingers wrapped around the top of the foot, place your left thumb onto the adrenal point. Use your right hand to flex the foot onto your left thumb and rotate the foot around the thumb.

USES: all nervous disorders, inflammatory conditions particularly rheumatoid arthritis, allergies especially asthma, lack of energy and exhaustion, pain relief.

BELOW THE WAISTLINE

STEP 17   RIGHT KIDNEY/URETER TUBE/BLADDER

Part of the kidney is located just above the waistline between zones 2 and 3. However the other half of the kidney, ureter tube and bladder are located below the waistline. After you have gently rotated the adrenal reflex move the thumb down slightly and you will have found the kidney reflex point. With the tip of your thumb pointing towards the toes press into the area and circle your thumb gently over the kidney area several times.

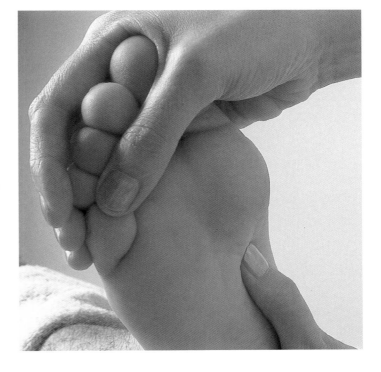

Turn the thumb around so that it is facing downwards then caterpillar walk down the ureter reflex towards the inside of the foot where the bladder reflex is situated beneath the inner ankle bone.

The bladder area can often look slightly puffy. You may either thumb walk or rotate on the bladder reflex.

USES: bladder infections, cystitis, fluid retention, bed wetting, incontinence.

STEP 18   SMALL INTESTINES

Hold the right foot back with your left hand and caterpillar walk
in horizontal rows from just below the waistline to the pelvic floor
line from the medial aspect (inside) of the foot as far as zone four.
You may work the whole of this area with your right thumb.

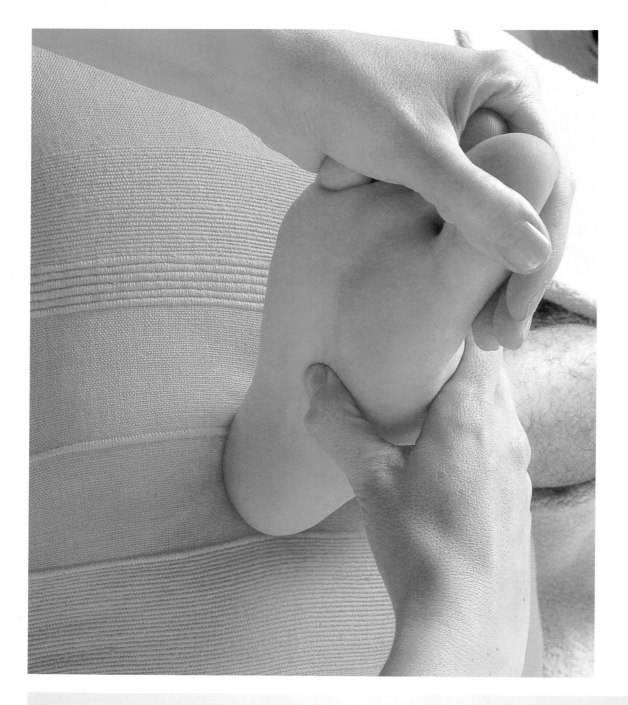

USES: digestive problems, abdominal cramps

STEP 19   ILEOCAECAL VALVE/ASCENDING AND TRANSVERSE COLON

The colon wraps around the small intestine. To locate the ileocaecal valve run your finger along zone five down the lower third of the sole of the foot towards the heel. Just above the pelvic floor line the hollow spot that you may feel is the ileocaecal valve reflex point. Using your left thumb press onto the point and circle several times over the reflex area.

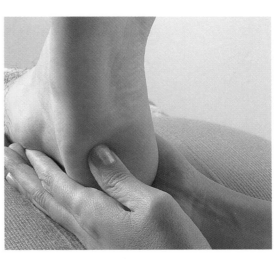

Then caterpillar walk with your left thumb up the ascending colon in zone 5 towards the waistline. You may feel a swelling either on or just below the waistline which is the hepatic flexure. Circle over this area several times.

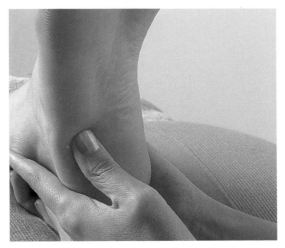

Then turn the thumb ninety degrees to the right and caterpillar walk horizontally along the transverse colon reflex following the waistline until you reach the inside of the sole of the foot.

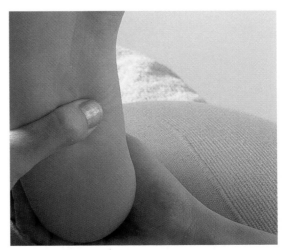

USES: constipation, diarrhoea, irritable bowel syndrome.

STEP 20 RIGHT SHOULDER/ARM/ELBOW/HAND/HIP/KNEE/LEG (OUTER EDGE OF THE FOOT)

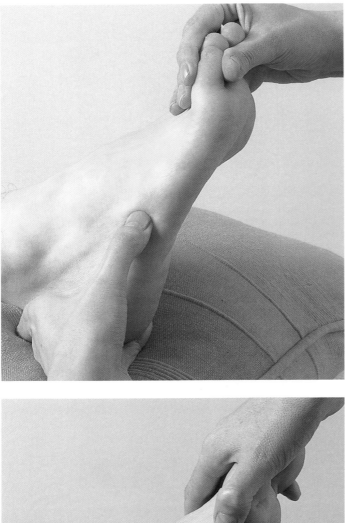

The areas corresponding to the joints of the body are situated along the outer edge of the foot. (Remember the spine runs the length of the inside of the foot).

Hold the toes of the right foot with your right hand and with your left thumb caterpillar walk vertically up the outer edge of the foot from the heel area up to the little toe.

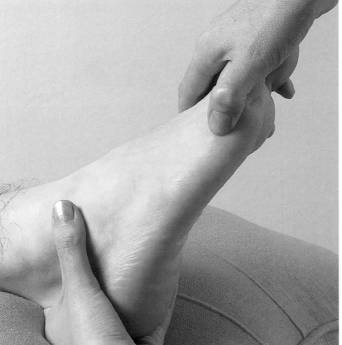

If you wish you may cup the right heel with your left hand and repeat the thumb walking in the opposite direction from the little toe to the heel. If you come across any areas that are tender then gently circle your thumb over them several times. The shoulder reflex on the bony prominence at the base of the little toe is likely to need attention.

Alternatively you may use your index finger to cover this area.

USES: all joint problems including arthritis, sports injuries, tennis elbow, frozen shoulder and housemaid's knee.

STEP 21 SCIATIC NERVE LINE/PELVIC AREA

The area around the Achilles tendon is not only worked for problems with the sciatic nerve but also for chronic ailments related to the prostate, uterus and the rectum.

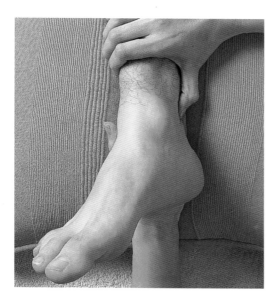

Hold the right foot with your left hand and place your right thumb approximately six inches above the inner ankle bone. Thumb walk down the Achilles tendon area towards the heel.

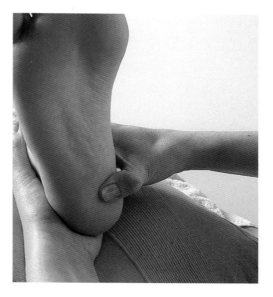

Continue to thumb walk across the sciatic nerve line on the hard heel pad of the right foot.

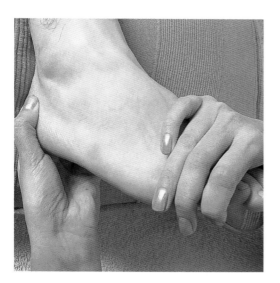

Finger walk or thumb walk up the outside of the foot along the Achilles tendon, changing hands if necessary.

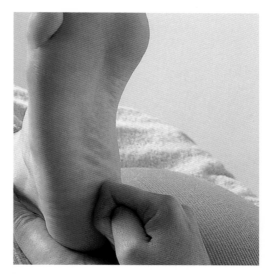

When there are problems with the pelvis it is very effective to work across the heel pad. Cup the foot with your left hand and gently work the area with your knuckles in a circular direction.

USES: sciatica, low back and hip problems, chronic problems with uterus, prostate and rectum

STEP 22 PROSTATE/UTERUS (BELOW INSIDE OF ANKLE)

All the reproductive organ reflexes are situated around the ankle area. To locate the prostate/uterus point place the index finger on the inner ankle bone and the third finger on the tip of the heel. Imagine a straight line running between your two fingers. The prostate/uterus lies in the middle of this imaginary line. Place the index finger onto the point and perform small circular pressure circles on the area.

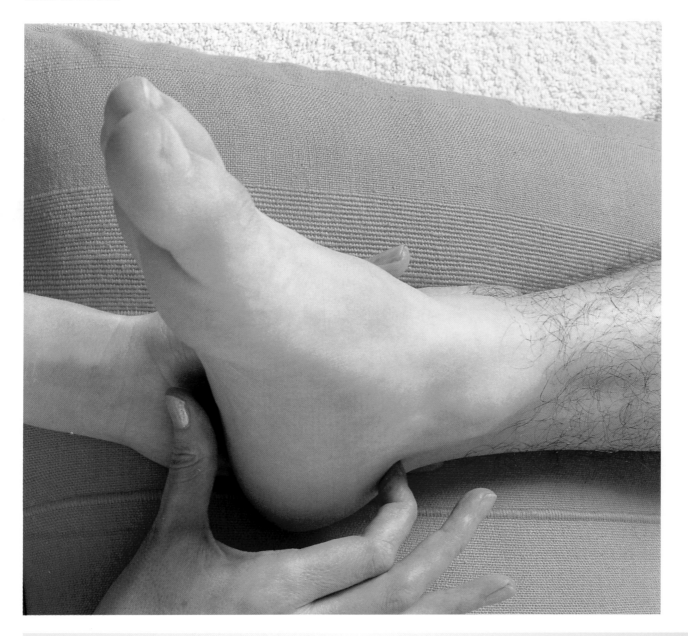

USES: all menstrual problems, painful, irregular periods, scanty or heavy menstruation, fertility problems, PMT, menopause, prostate problems,.

STEP 23 VAS DEFERENS/LYMPH/GROIN/FALLOPIAN TUBE (ACROSS THE TOP OF THE FOOT)

Thumb walk or finger walk from the inside of the ankle across the top of the foot to the outside of the ankle. This area should be walked in both directions.

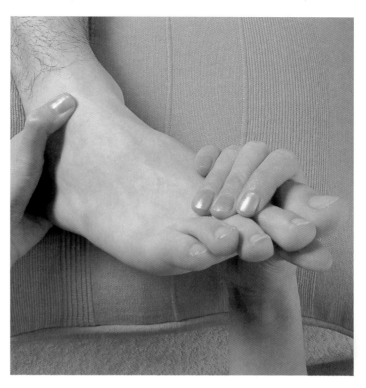

It can be quite a sensitive area – remember if you find a tender area gently massage it in a circular direction.

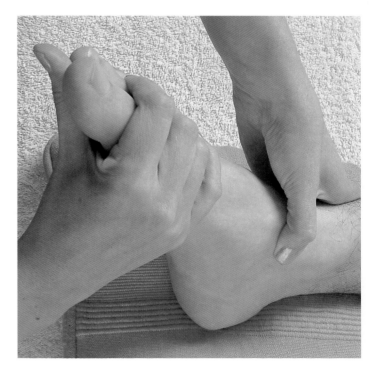

USES: problems with the male or female reproductive organs, swelling of the feet.
Toxins are drained and the immune system is boosted.

STEP 24 RIGHT TESTICLE/OVARY (BELOW OUTSIDE OF ANKLE)

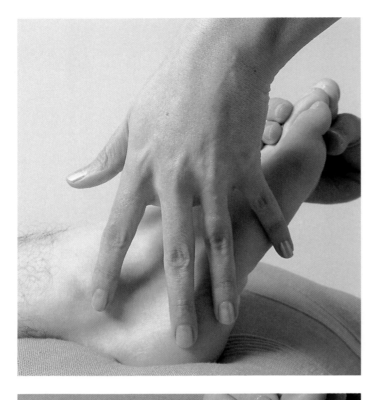

Locate the testicle/ovary reflex by drawing an imaginary diagonal line from the outer ankle bone to the top of the heel and finding the mid-point.

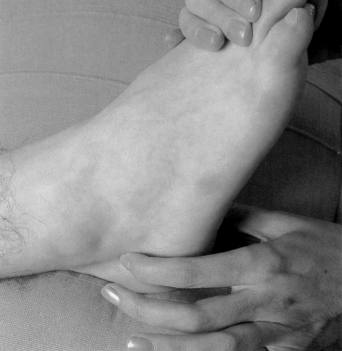

Now you should perform small circular movements over this area with your index finger.

USES: infertility problems, menstrual irregularities, ovarian cysts, menopause.

STEP 25   COMPLETING THE RIGHT FOOT

Using both hands, stroke the whole foot working up from the toes gliding around the ankle bones and back again. These stroking movements should ensure that any toxins which have been released during the reflexology sequence are dispersed and totally relax the right foot. Now cover up the right foot.

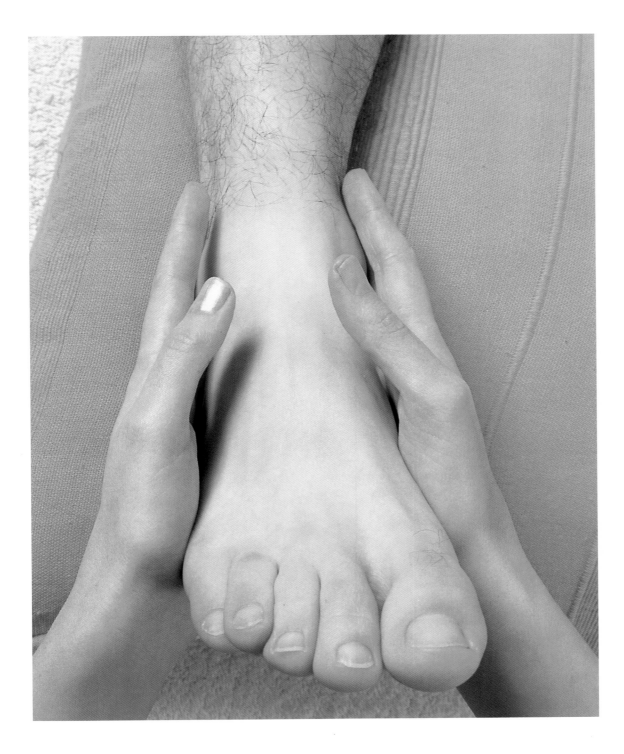

RELAXATION TECHNIQUES

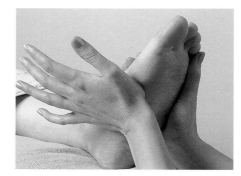

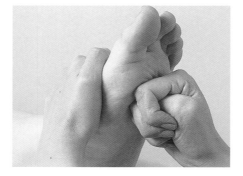
Effleurage/stroking

Metatarsal kneading

Alternate thumb rotations

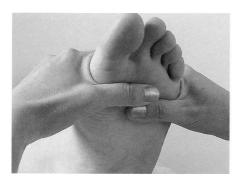
Zig-zag/spreading the foot

Spinal stroking

Spinal twist

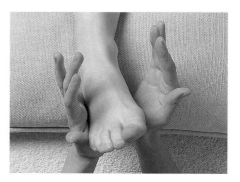

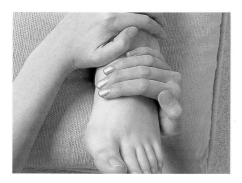
Toe loosening

Ankle rotations

Foot rocking

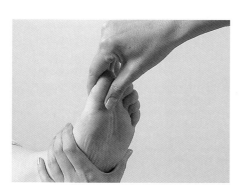

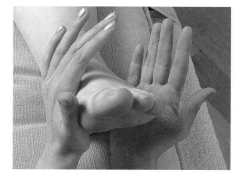

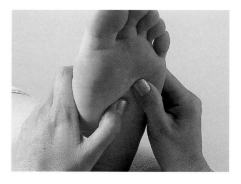

TENSION RELEASE

STEP 1 DIAPHRAGM/SOLAR PLEXUS

To locate the solar plexus and diaphragm, gently pull the toes backwards with your left hand. Hold the toes with your thumb on the sole of the foot, fingers on the top.

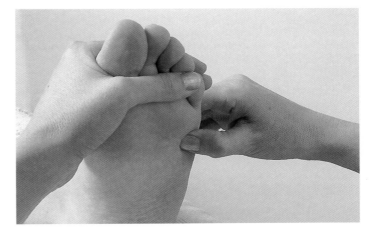

Walk across the diaphragm line with your right thumb working from the outside of the foot towards the inside.

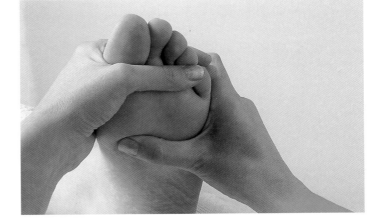

When you reach the solar plexus press gently into it is as the receiver breathes in and release the pressure as they breathe out. Repeat several times.

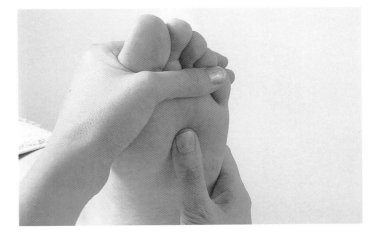

USES: relaxation and release of tension

HEAD AND NECK AREA

STEP 2 HEAD AND BRAIN AREA (BACK AND SIDES OF THE BIG TOE)

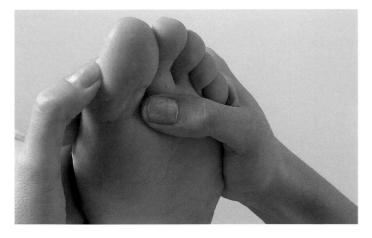

Wrap the fingers of your right hand over the front of the toes with your thumb under the back of the toes. Using your left thumb walk from the outer edge of the base of the big toe.

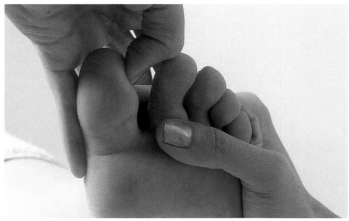

Now continue walking up the outside of the toe, over the top and finally down the inside.

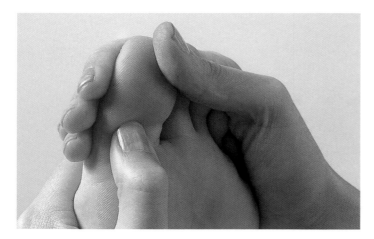

With your left thumb walk up the back of the big toe from the base to the tip several times to cover the whole area.

USES: Working the head and brain is particularly useful for conditions such as headaches and migraine. Also for any problems affecting the brain such as defects in memory, lack of concentration or inability to think clearly.

STEP 3   PITUITARY GLAND (BIG TOE)

To locate the pituitary gland find the widest point of the big toe and draw an imaginary line. The pituitary gland is approximately in the middle of this line but remember you often have to search for it. Place the fingers of your right hand over the front of the toes and your thumb under the back of the toes. Using the hook-in and back-up technique press the pituitary gland with the corner of your left thumb.

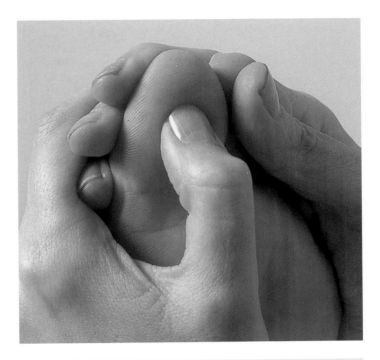

USES: All hormonal problems. (This point is often out of balance)

STEP 4   FACE (FRONT OF THE BIG TOE)

Wrap your left hand around the top of the foot just below the base of the toes, left thumb under the sole of the foot, fingers on the top. Use your right index finger to walk down the front of the big toe from the tip to the base until the whole of the area has been covered. You may also use your index and middle finger if you are very coordinated.

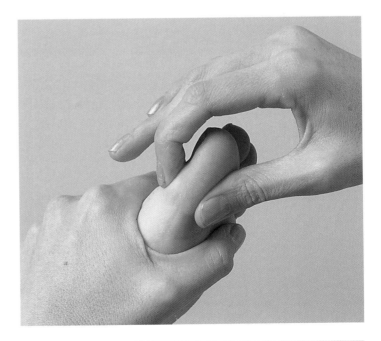

USES: Any facial problems, e.g. neuralgia, eye, nose, mouth, teeth, gum and jaw problems.

STEP 5 NECK (BASE OF THE BIG TOE)

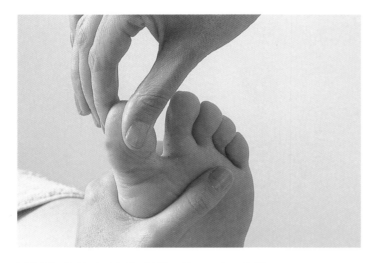

Support the left foot with your left hand and grasp the big toe between your right thumb and forefinger. Rotate the big toe clockwise and anti-clockwise to improve the mobility of the neck.

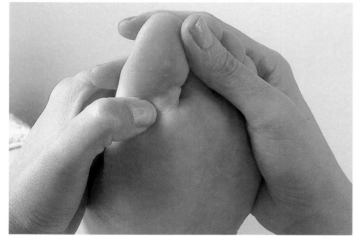

Now wrap your right hand around the top of the foot, fingers on the top, thumb on the sole. Walk across the back of the base of the big toe using your left thumb.

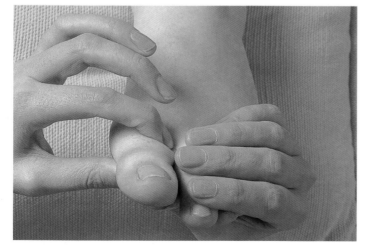

Use your index finger to walk across the base of the front of the toe working from outside to inside.

USES: All neck disorders, problems with the throat, tonsils and vocal chords, thyroid and parathyroid.

STEP 6   SINUSES (BACK, SIDES AND TOP OF THE SMALL TOES)

Support the left foot between the thumb and fingers of your right hand, thumb on the sole of the foot, fingers over the front of the toes. With your left thumb use very small caterpillar steps to walk from the top to the base of each toe.

Use your left thumb, index finger or thumb and index finger together to walk down the sides of each toe. If you prefer you may walk up the toes instead of down but it is often more effective to work down the toes. It also makes more sense as you are draining towards the lymph glands.

USES: sinus problems, headaches caused by sinus congestion, hay fever, catarrh and allergies.

STEP 7   TEETH (FRONT OF THE TOES)

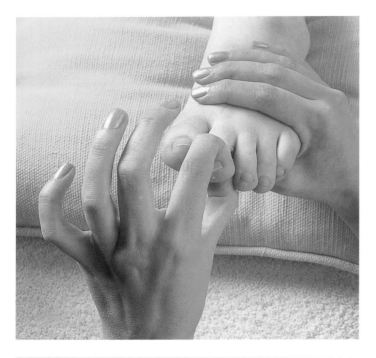

Wrap your right hand around the top of the foot. Commencing at the base of the nail finger walk with your left index finger down the fronts of the small toes.

USES: toothache, sensitive, painful or infected gums.

STEP 8   UPPER LYMPHATICS (BETWEEN THE TOES)

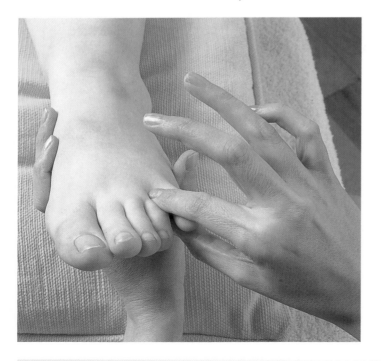

Support the foot with your left hand. Use the thumb and finger of your right hand to gently squeeze the webbing between each of the toes.

USES: to fight off and to prevent any infections.

STEP 9 SPINE (INNER EDGE OF THE FOOT)

Cup the heel of the left foot with your left hand. Using your right thumb caterpillar walk down the inside of the foot from the base of the big toenail to the heel. (Sequence 1–3) If you feel any gritty or tender areas gently massage the crystals away.

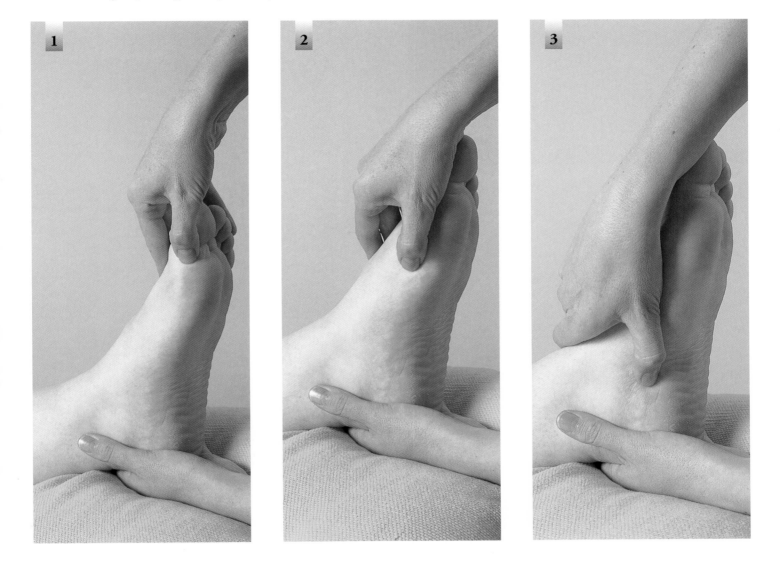

You may also walk in the opposite direction from the heel to the base of the toenail.

USES: All back problems, lack of mobility, arthritis, disc problems. Pain and stiffness should be greatly reduced.

STEP 10 EYES AND EARS (BASE OF THE TOES)

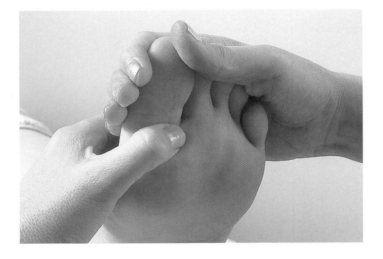

Pull the toes gently back with your holding hand and thumb walk across the ridge at the base of the toes in both directions.

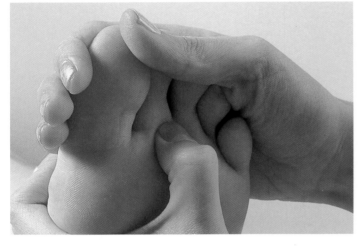

To locate the left eye point walk across the base of the toes and stop between the second and third toes. Press firmly into this point using the hook in and back-up technique.

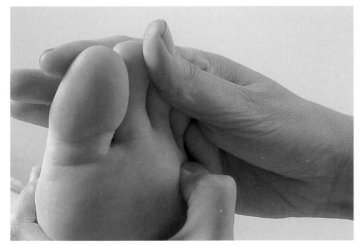

To find the left ear point continue your caterpillar walk as far as between the fourth and fifth toes. Use the hook in and back-up technique on this area.

USES: sore, tired or watery eyes, glaucoma, conjunctivitis and eyesight problems.
Earache, glue ear, tinnitus, hearing problems, vertigo and dizziness.

SHOULDER GIRDLE LINE TO DIAPHRAGM LINE

STEP 11 THYROID/PARATHYROID/THYMUS

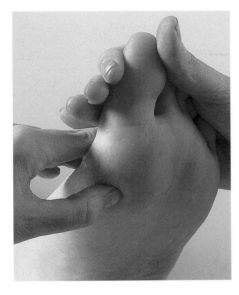

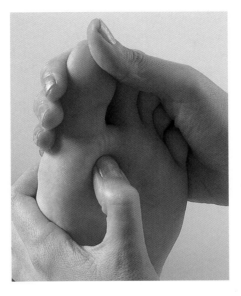

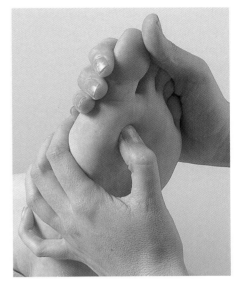

Support the toes with your right hand. Place your left thumb below the ball on the diaphragm line just on the inside of the foot.

Walk in a curved direction up to between the big and the second toe. Caterpillar walk the pad under the big toe until you have completely covered the area.

Find the thyroid point in the centre of the pad of the ball of the foot below the big toe. Place your left thumb onto the thyroid reflex and circle gently over the area several times.

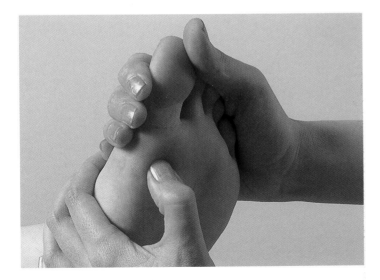

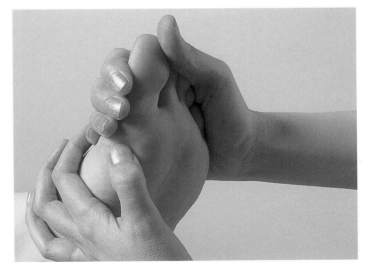

Move your left thumb over to the right to contact the parathyroid area and perform pressure circles on this area.

Slide your left thumb over towards the inside of the foot and rotate it gently over the thymus point.

USES: thyroid problems, weight problems, nervousness, palpitations, dry skin, lethargy, menopause.
The thymus gland is important to maintain a healthy immune system

STEP 12   LEFT LUNG/CHEST (BALL OF THE FOOT)

To treat to the left lung you will work across the entire area from the shoulder girdle line to the diaphragm line. Pull the toes back with your right hand fingers wrapped around the front of the foot thumb underneath. With your left thumb walk in vertical strips from the diaphragm line to the shoulder girdle line. (Sequence 1–2).

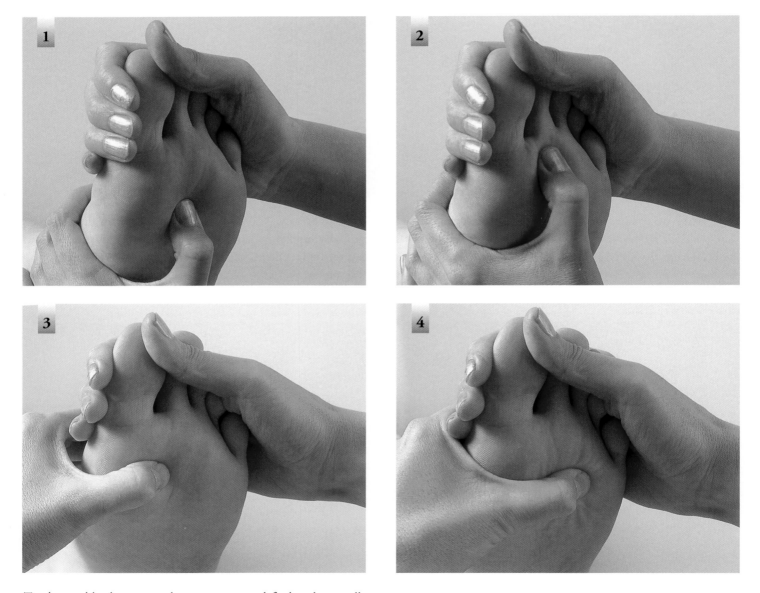

To thoroughly de-congest the area use your left thumb to walk across the area in horizontal strips (Sequence 3–4).

USES: coughs and colds, asthma, bronchitis, emphysema, shallow breathing, hyperventilation and panic attacks.

STEP 13 LEFT LUNG/BREAST/MAMMARY GLANDS (TOP OF THE FOOT)

Pull all the toes very GENTLY back towards you with your left hand, fingers on top of the foot, thumb underneath. Use your right index finger or your index and middle finger to walk down the front of the foot in vertical strips as far as the diaphragm line.

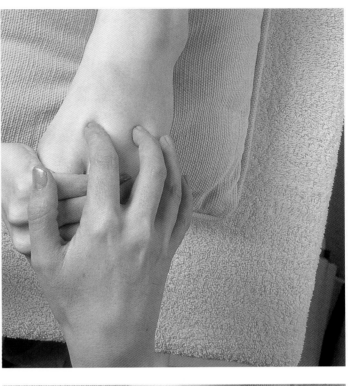

Alternatively make a fist with one of your hands and place it under the toes as a support. Now finger walk the lung/breast area in the same way as shown in previous step.

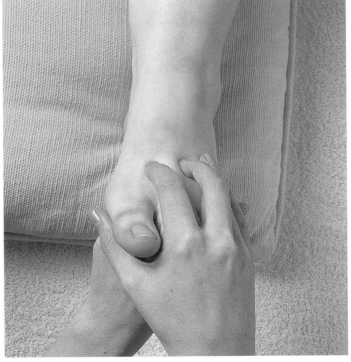

USES: respiratory problems as described in step twelve, breast problems such as tenderness due to P.M.T, harmless lumps which have been investigated

STEP 14   HEART AREA

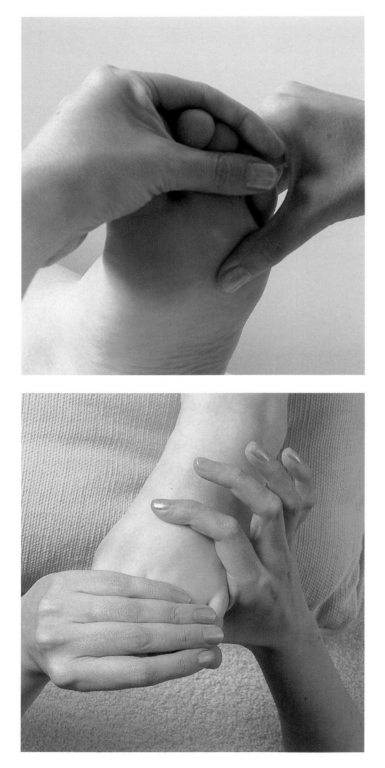

Hold the foot in your left hand and wrap your right hand over the foot, thumb on the sole, fingers on the top. Gently massage with your right thumb the upper third of the sole of the foot from the shoulder girdle line to the diaphragm line working in a circular direction.

Now repeat these movements using your right index finger on the top of the foot. As you work the heart area you will also be working the left lung as these two reflexes overlap considerably.

The heart is located mostly on the left foot between the shoulder girdle line and the diaphragm line. If any pain or sensitivity is felt in this area then do NOT increase your pressure. Deep pressure should NEVER be used on this area immediately after a heart attack or if a pacemaker has been fitted.

USES: to regulate the heartbeat, palpitations and to promote an easier flow of blood to the heart.

DIAPHRAGM LINE TO WAISTLINE

STEP 15   STOMACH/PANCREAS/DUODENUM

Hold the foot in the right hand, thumb on the sole, fingers on the top. Place your thumb just below the inside edge of the diaphragm line. Thumb walk in horizontal rows from zone one to zone four until the entire area from diaphragm line to waistline has been covered.

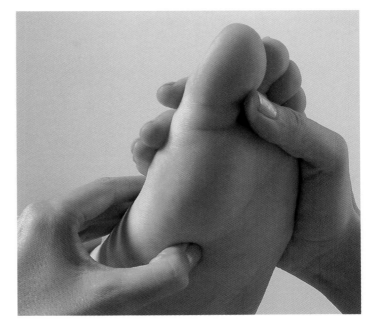

USES: stomach problems such as indigestion, hyperacidity, ulcers and stomach cramps

STEP 16   SPLEEN

To treat the spleen which is ONLY found on the left foot, hold the foot with your left hand. Place your right thumb just below the outside edge of the diaphragm line and caterpillar walk from zone five to zone four in horizontal rows.

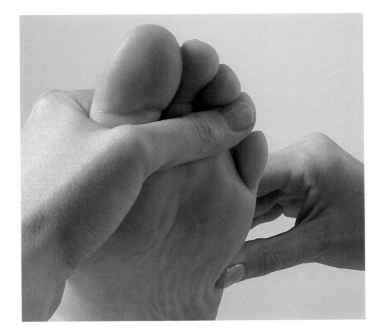

USES: to treat when the immune system is low or to combat infections

STEP 17   LEFT ADRENAL GLAND

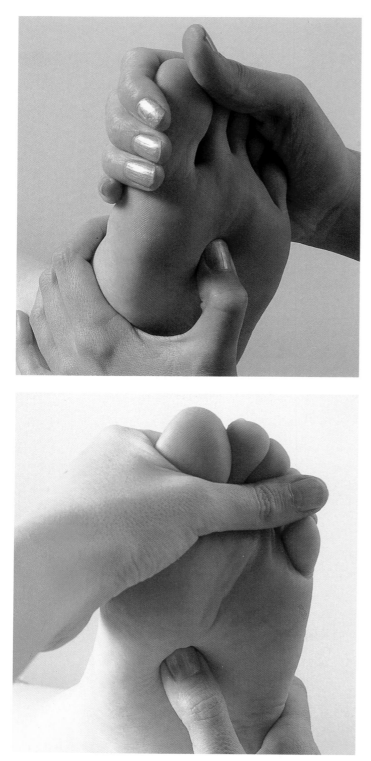

To locate the adrenal gland, pull back the toes until a thick tendon protrudes which runs from the big toe to the heel. The reflex point is found midway between the diaphragm and waistlines on the inside of this tendon. Hold the left foot with your left hand, place your right thumb onto the adrenal point.

Use your left hand to flex the foot onto your right thumb and rotate the foot around thumb.

USES: all nervous disorders, inflammatory conditions particularly rheumatoid arthritis, allergies especially asthma, lack of energy and exhaustion, pain relief.

BELOW THE WAISTLINE

STEP 18   LEFT KIDNEY/URETER/BLADDER

After you have gently treated the left adrenal gland move your right thumb down slightly. With the pad of your right thumb pointing towards the toes press into the area and circle it gently over the kidney area several times.

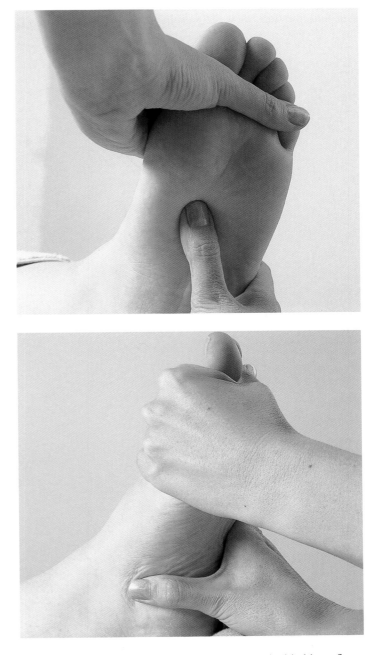

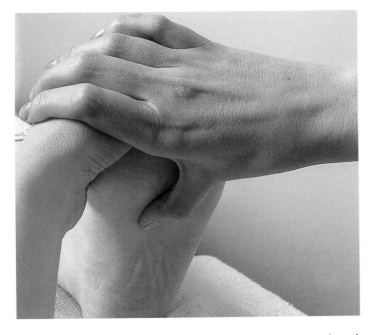

Now turn your thumb around so that it is facing downwards and caterpillar walk down the ureter reflex towards the inside of the foot – the bladder reflex is found beneath the inner ankle bone.

Either thumb walk over this point or rotate on the bladder reflex.

USES: bladder infections, cystitis, fluid retention, bed wetting, incontinence.

STEP 19 SMALL INTESTINES

Hold the left foot back with your right hand and with your left
thumb walk in horizontal rows from the inside the foot as far as
zone four from just below the waistline to the pelvic floor line.

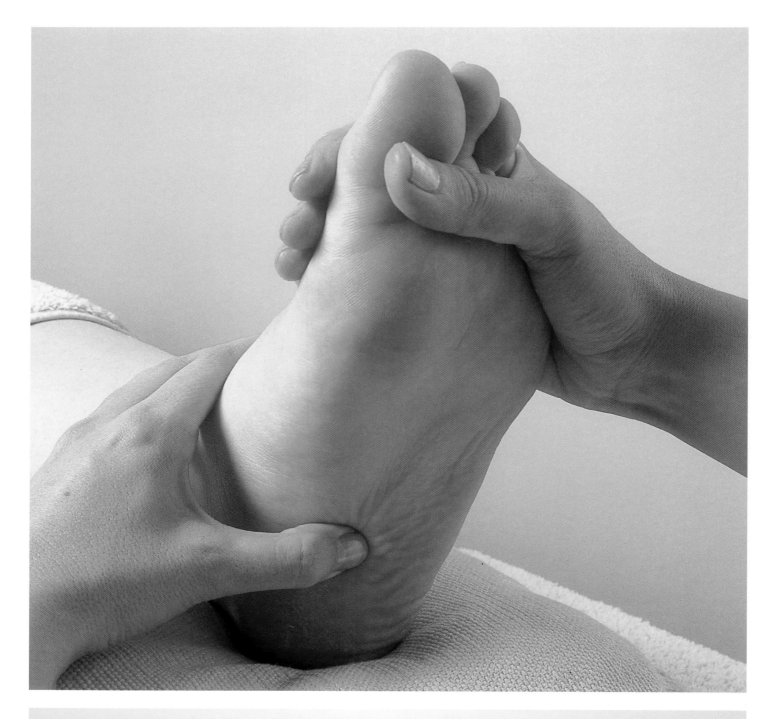

USES: digestive problems, abdominal cramps

STEP 20 TRANSVERSE COLON/DESCENDING COLON/SIGMOID COLON

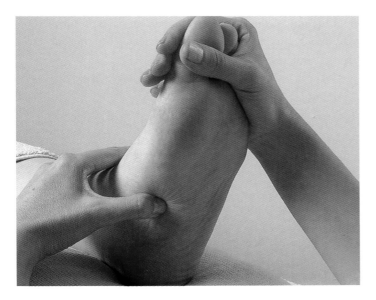

Hold the toes of the left foot in your right hand. Place your left thumb just below the waistline on the inner side of the sole of the foot.

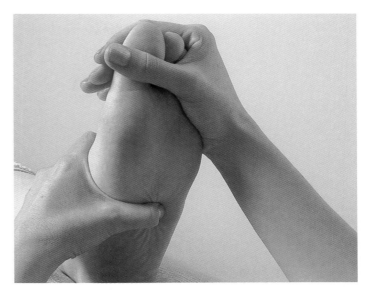

Caterpillar walk across the transverse colon following the waistline until you reach zone five on the outer edge of the left foot.

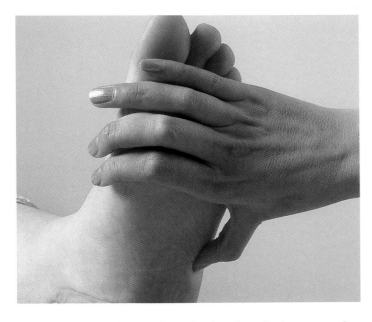

Change hands and using the right thumb walk down zone five which is the descending colon towards the heel.

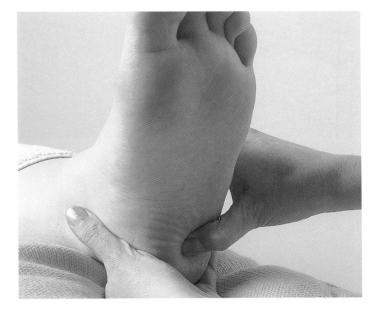

Just before you reach the pelvic floor line turn the right thumb 45° diagonally to the left until you reach the sciatic line. Swivel the right thumb round and circle several times to treat to the sigmoid colon. Then continue caterpillar walking towards the bladder area.

USES: constipation, diarrhoea, irritable bowel syndrome.

STEP 21 LEFT SHOULDER/ARM/ELBOW/HAND/HIP/KNEE/LEG (OUTER EDGE OF THE FOOT)

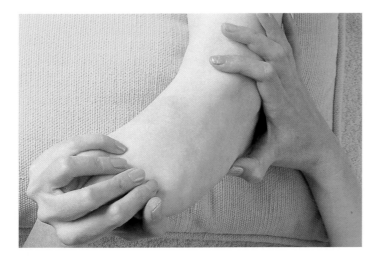

Hold the toes of the left foot with your left hand and with your right thumb caterpillar walk along the outer edge of the foot.

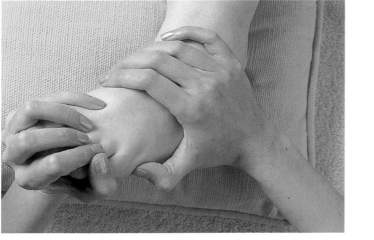

Continue caterpillar walking until you have covered the whole area from the heel to the little toe,

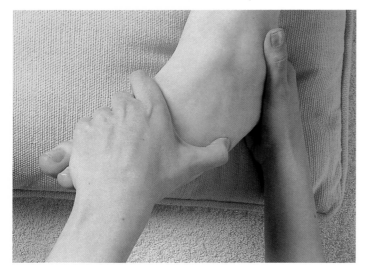

Now cup the left heel with your right hand and walk your left thumb in the opposite direction from the little toe to the heel.

USES: all joint problems including arthritis, sports injuries, tennis elbow, frozen shoulder and housemaid's knee.

STEP 22 SCIATIC NERVE LINE/PELVIC AREA

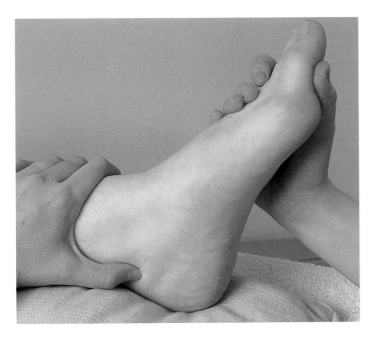

Hold the ball of the left foot with your right hand and place your left thumb about six inches above the inner heel bone. thumb walk down the Achilles tendon towards the heel.

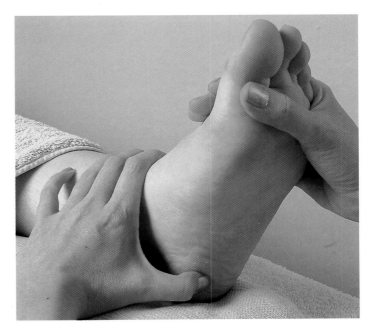

Continue to walk across the hard heel pad all along the sciatic nerve line.

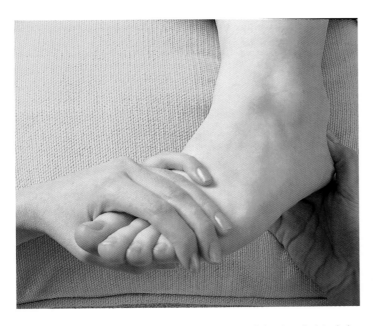

With your right thumb walk up the outside of the foot behind the ankle bone along the Achilles tendon.

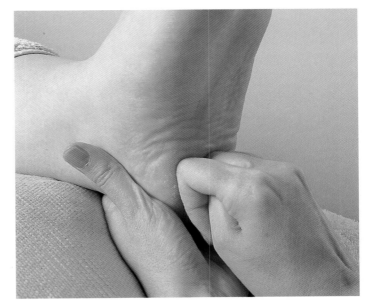

Now cup the foot with your left hand and work across the heel pad with your knuckles in a circular direction.

USES: sciatica, low back and hip problems, chronic problems with uterus, prostate and rectum

STEP 23 UTERUS/PROSTATE (BELOW INSIDE OF ANKLE)

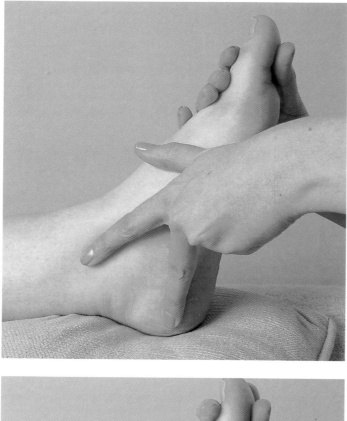

To pinpoint this reflex area place the index finger on the inner ankle bone and the third finger on the tip of the heel. Imagine a straight line running between your two fingers.

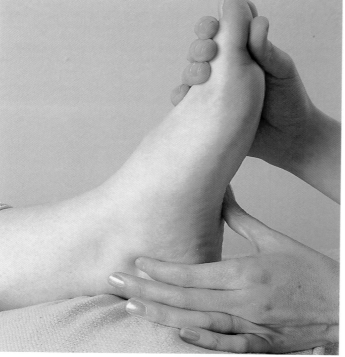

In the middle of this imaginary line is the uterus/prostate point. Place your index finger on this point and perform small circular pressure circles on this area.

USES: all menstrual problems, prostate problems, painful, irregular periods, scanty or heavy menstruation, fertility problems, PMT, menopause.

STEP 24 FALLOPIAN TUBE/VAS DEFERENS/LYMPH/GROIN (ACROSS THE TOP OF THE FOOT)

Using your left thumb walk from the inside of the ankle across the top of the foot to the outside of the ankle.

Now continue walking in the same direction.

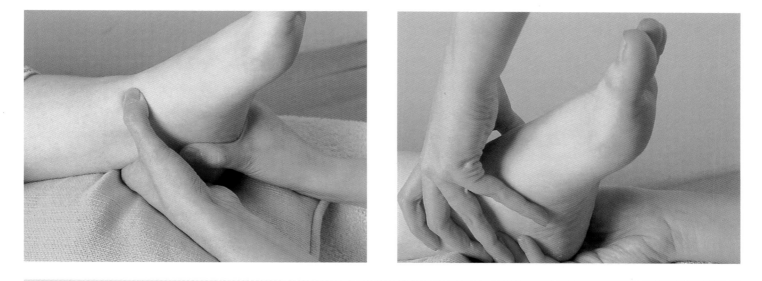

USES: problems with the male or female reproductive organs, swelling of the feet.
Toxins are drained and the immune system is boosted.

STEP 25 LEFT OVARY/TESTICLE (BELOW OUTSIDE OF THE ANKLE)

Draw an imaginary diagonal line from the outer ankle bone to the tip of the heel and find the mid-point. Now perform small circular movements all over this area using your right index finger.

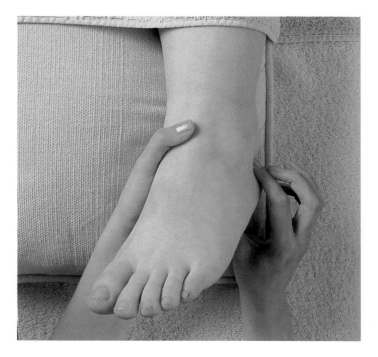

USES: infertility problems, menstrual irregularities, ovarian cysts, menopause.

STEP 26 COMPLETING THE LEFT FOOT

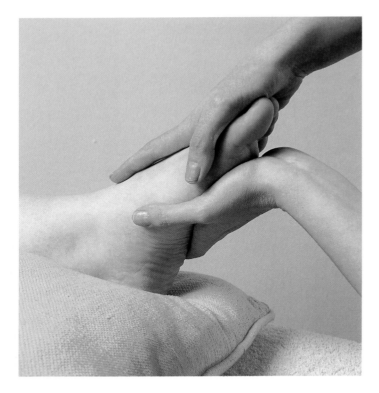

To completely disperse any toxins which have been released during the treatment stroke the left foot from the toes up to the ankle bones and back again as many times as you like.

Well done. You have now completed both feet.

THE FINALE

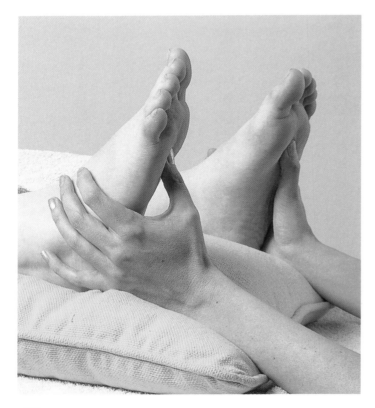

1. Uncover both feet and return to any reflex points that were tender during the reflexology session in order to give them further attention.

2. Use any of your favourite relaxation techniques.

3. Very gently and lightly run your fingertips down the tops and sides of the feet barely touching the skin.

4. To complete your reflexology session carry out the solar plexus release. Place both thumbs into the hollows on the soles of the feet at the diaphragm line. Press gently and slowly into the solar plexus reflex points as the recipient breathes in. Gradually release your pressure as he/she breathes out.

5. Cover the feet up and leave the recipient to relax for while.

6. When they get up give them a large glass of water to drink and encourage them to drink plenty of water over the next 24 hours to flush out the toxins.

reflexology for
Common Ailments

MAIN TREATMENTS

During a reflexology session, tender areas may indicate certain imbalances. After a treatment you can come back to these tender areas to give them more attention.

This section looks at some common ailments, and suggests areas to concentrate on. Many of these areas feature in all or most of the recommended treatments. These are illustrated here. Other, specific areas are illustrated throughout the section. If you are uncertain of any point, please refer back to these pages.

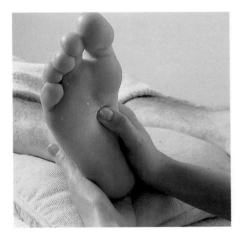

Adrenals

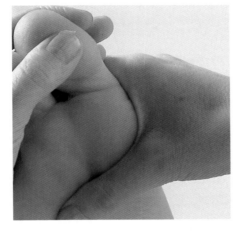

Diaphragm

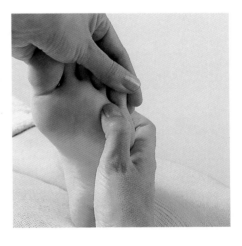

Ears

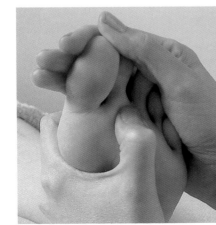

Eyes

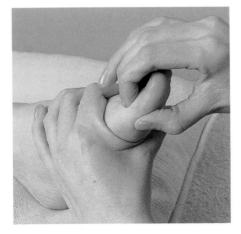

Face

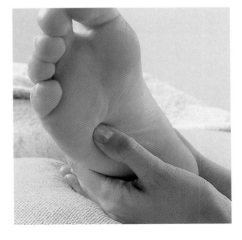

Gallbladder

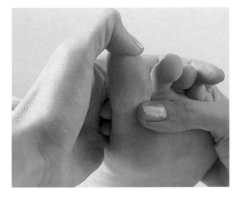

Head and brain

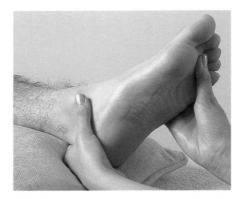

Heart area

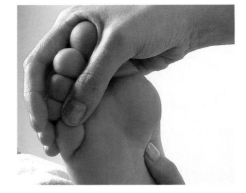

Kidneys

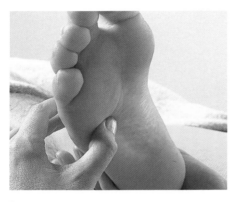

Liver

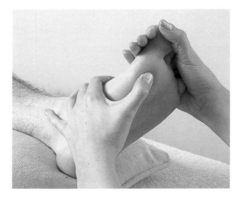

Lung/chest area

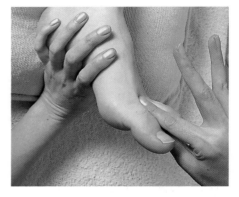

Upper Lymphatics

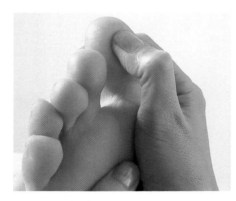

Pituitary gland

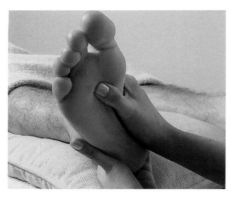

Solar Plexus

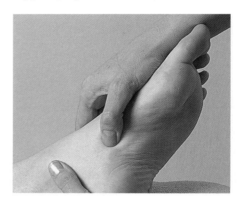

Spine

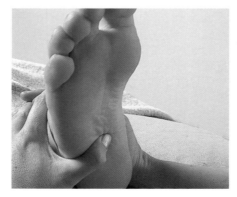

Transverse colon

CIRCULATORY PROBLEMS

Heart disease is one of the main causes of premature death in the developed countries. Contributory factors include poor diet, obesity, high stress levels, lack of exercise, genetic predisposition and smoking. Reflexology is excellent for improving the circulation, balancing the blood pressure and reducing stress on the heart.

ANGINA

Angina is caused by a lack of oxygen reaching the heart muscle usually as a result of hardening of the arteries. Chest pain is experienced due to the decreased blood and oxygen supply to the heart tissue.

Causes
- high fat diet
- stress
- lack of exercise
- hereditary factors
- smoking

Other advice
- eat a healthy diet — avoid junk food, sugar and salt, fried foods and saturated animal fats. Instead eat plenty of fresh fruit and vegetables, fibre and virgin olive oil
- give up smoking
- take regular, gentle physical exercise – e.g. a 20 minutes walk daily, Tai Chi or yoga

Reflexology Treatment

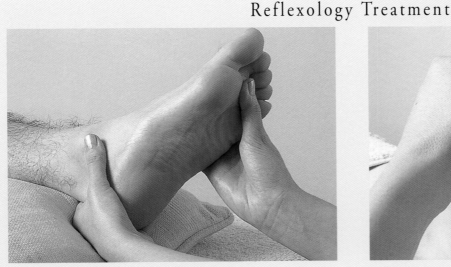

Heart area

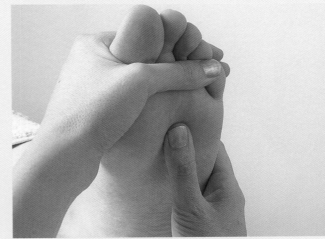

Solar Plexus

- Heart area
- Liver – to help normalise cholesterol
- Adrenals – to relieve stress
- Solar plexus
- Diaphragm — to deepen breathing
- Lungs and chest – to relax and open up chest area

HYPERTENSION (HIGH BLOOD PRESSURE)

High blood pressure is a fairly common disorder which increases with age. Hypertension, if left untreated, can result in heart and kidney failure or strokes.

Causes

- stress
- obesity
- smoking
- family history

Other advice

- avoid salt, sugar and saturated fats
- eat lots of fruit, vegetables, fibre (especially oats) and garlic
- give up smoking and reduce alcohol and caffeine intake
- reduce stress
- take gentle, regular exercise

Reflexology Treatment

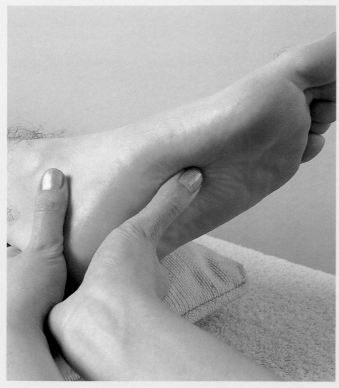

Kidneys

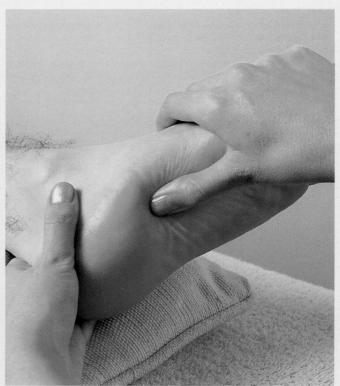

Working from the kidney towards the bladder

- Heart area
- Kidneys
- Adrenal glands – to reduce stress
- Solar plexus
- Diaphragm – to deepen breathing
- Lungs and chest – to relax the chest area

DIGESTIVE PROBLEMS

The majority of people suffer at some time from a digestive disorder. The digestive system is very prone to upset particularly by stress. Imbalance can be caused by emotions such as anger, tension and fear or by eating food too quickly. Many of us snack on junk foods and refined foods with little nutritional value which also may contain harmful colourings and preservatives.

We also drink far too much tea, coffee and soft carbonated drinks with caffeine in them. Our bodies would prefer 6-8 glasses of water a day!

Reflexology is an excellent tool for releasing tension and aiding the process of digestion and elimination.

A doctor should of course always be consulted for any digestive problem if it is persistent or accompanied by weight loss, blood in the faeces or a general sense of being unwell.

INDIGESTION/HEARTBURN (DYSPEPSIA)

Causes

- excessive eating and drinking, rushing or not chewing food properly
- eating the wrong foods e.g. dairy foods, refined foods such as cakes and biscuits, fatty foods, hot and spicy or rich foods
- stress which increases stomach acid

Other advice

- avoid stressful situations
- reduce foods that cause heartburn

Reflexology Treatment

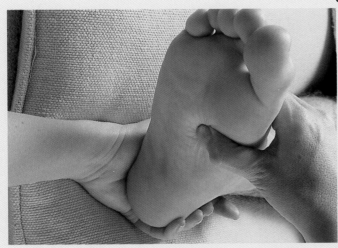

Stomach/pancreas/duodenum

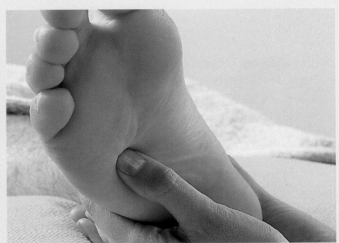

Liver/gallbladder

- Stomach/pancreas/duodenum
- Liver/gallbladder – if there is nausea
- Solar plexus – to reduce tension
- Adrenal gland – to reduce inflammation

CONSTIPATION

Causes

- poor diet and inadequate intake of water
- lack of exercise
- tension
- certain drugs such as too many laxatives which make the bowel lazy, antibiotics, pain killers, steroids and diuretics

IRRITABLE BOWEL SYNDROME

This disorder is becoming increasingly prevalent and is characterised by pain in the abdominal area which can be very intense and a combination of constipation and diarrhoea.

Causes

- stress is a major trigger of irritable bowel syndrome
- certain types of foods which can cause an attack vary enormously but common culprits include dairy foods, wheat, chocolate, coffee and alcohol

Reflexology Treatment

- Small intestines
- Ileocaecal valve, which controls movement between the small and large intestines
- Large intestines:
  - ascending colon
  - transverse (right foot) colon
  - transverse (left foot) colon
  - descending colon
- Chronic rectum
- Solar plexus – to reduce tension

For irritable bowel syndrome only:
- Adrenals – to reduce inflammation and irritation within the digestive tract

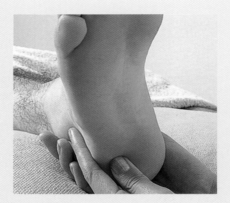

Ileocaecal valve

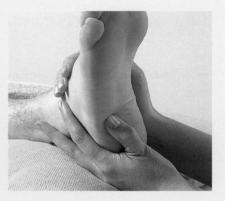

Ascending colon

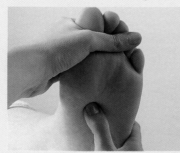

Adrenals

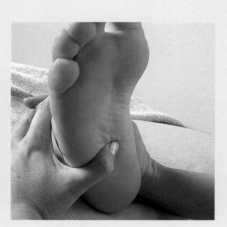

Transverse colon

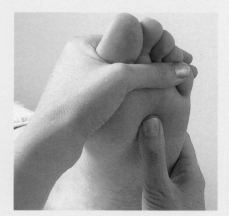

Solar Plexus

Other advice

- avoid stress
- eat a healthy high fibre diet to increase the frequency and quantity of bowel movements
- drink 6 – 8 glasses of water per day
- do not ignore the urge to move your bowels
- avoid prolonged use of laxatives which can make the bowel lazy

LIVER/GALLBLADDER PROBLEMS

NB. The gallbladder should always be treated with care. Never massage the gallbladder vigorously where there are gallstones. Gentle reflexology on this area however is often very successful: certain patients awaiting operations have had their gallstones eliminated with the aid of reflexology. Gallstones are formed from cholesterol, bile pigments and calcium compounds. They can cause colicky pain when found in the gallbladder (although only about 20% of gallstones cause symptoms). If they are found in the bile ducts (which connect the gallbladder and liver to the duodenum) then the pain can be excruciating.

Causes
- fatty diet
- obesity

Other advice
- eat a low fat, low sugar diet
- increase fibre in the diet
- drink fresh lemon squeezed into warm water
- eat celery

Reflexology Treatment

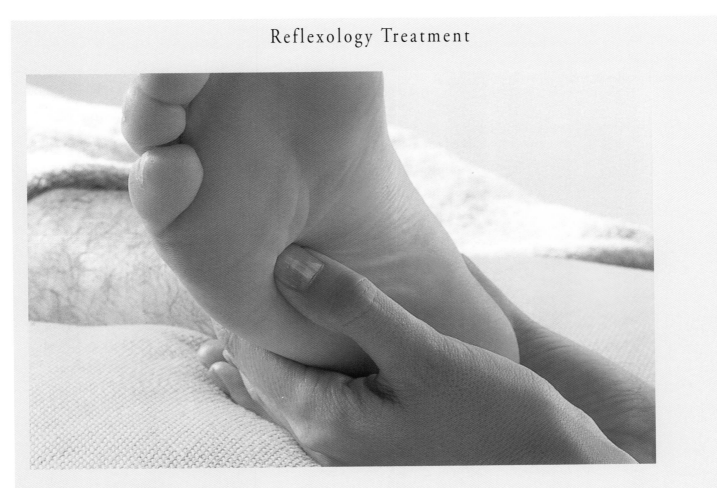

Liver

- Liver
- Gallbladder

GENITO-URINARY PROBLEMS

Women particularly can suffer from a whole host of conditions as the hormones are so easily unbalanced. Reflexology is excellent for relieving both the physical and emotional symptoms which can occur.

CYSTITIS

Cystitis is an inflammation of the inner lining of the bladder giving rise to frequent urination, burning or stinging sensations, low backache and a feeling of being run down.

Causes
- infection passing from the urethral opening into the bladder. The bacteria can come from the vagina or from the intestines via the anus
- stress often precedes an attack

NB always work FROM the kidney towards the bladder. NEVER go back up – otherwise you could transfer the infection. A kidney infection is much more serious than a bladder infection.

Other advice
- drink cranberry juice
- increase fluid intake to flush out the bladder

Reflexology Treatment

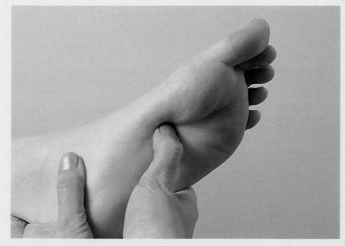

Adrenals

Bladder

- Kidneys
- Bladder – which will often and look raised and puffy where there is an infection
- Lower spine – for pain relief
- Adrenals – for inflammation

MENSTRUAL PROBLEMS

These include pre-menstrual syndrome (PMS), painful periods, absent or scanty periods and the menopause. Reflexology can correct hormonal imbalances, relax the body and mind, give pain relief from menstrual cramps and aid the elimination of excess fluid from the body.

Causes
- hormonal imbalances
- stress
- change in menstrual cycle

Other advice
- reduce salt which leads to fluid retention
- reduce sugar and caffeine which aggravate mood swings
- increase fibre
- take a B -complex supplement
- gentle exercise such as yoga and Tai Chi
- if menopausal increase calcium rich foods – e.g. fish especially sardines, sunflower, pumpkin, sesame seeds and nuts

Reflexology Treatment

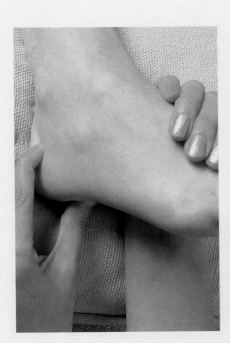

Ovaries

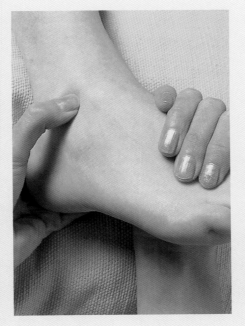

Fallopian Tubes

Breast area

- All reproductive areas:
  – Ovaries
  – Uterus
  – Fallopian tubes
- Kidneys – to remove excess fluid
- Breasts – to alleviate soreness
- Pituitary gland – to balance hormones
- Solar plexus – to relax
- Spine – to relieve back strain and cramps

HEAD AND NECK PROBLEMS

Common problems affecting this area include headaches, migraine and nasal problems such as catarrh, sinusitis and also hay fever.

HEADACHES/MIGRAINE

Most of us suffer from headaches at some time – the majority of which originate in the neck and shoulders. The really unlucky ones suffer from migraine, a one-sided headache characterised by intense pain and sometimes sickness and blurring of vision.

Causes

- anxiety
- tension in the neck
- hormonal imbalances
- irregular meals
- certain foods causing an allergic reaction
- tiredness and over use of the eyes

Other advice

- reduce stress
- if you suffer with migraine try avoiding chocolate, cheese, drinks with caffeine in especially coffee, alcohol especially red wine and food additives

Reflexology Treatment

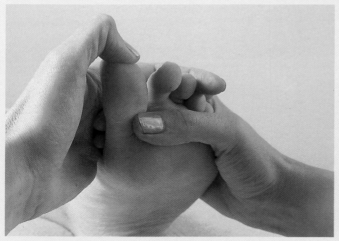

Head and Brain

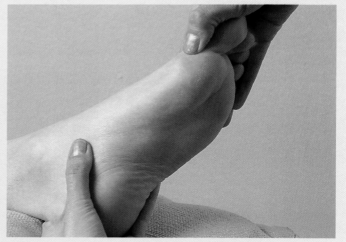

Spine

- Head and brain area
- Spine with emphasis on the neck area
- Pituitary gland – to balance the hormones
- Liver – to reduce toxicity and nausea (the entire digestive system may be worked to improve elimination)
- Eyes
- Solar plexus – to reduce stress and tension

NASAL PROBLEMS

Reflexology is excellent for nasal problems and in particular sinusitis and hay fever. Some sufferers find that regular treatment commencing a few months prior to the hay fever season is highly effective.

Causes
- infections and the after effects of a cold
- allergic responses e.g. to pollen/dust

Other advice
- avoid dairy foods which increase the production of mucus
- steam inhalations

Reflexology Treatment

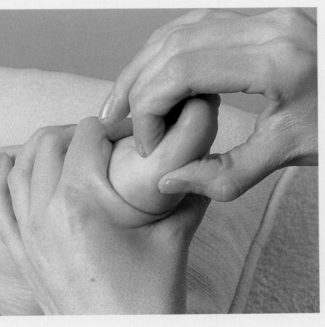

Face

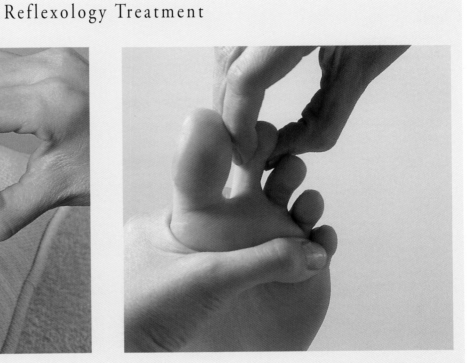

Sinuses

- Face area
- Sinuses
- Adrenals – to reduce inflammation
- Eyes
- Ears

MUSCULO-SKELETAL PROBLEMS

Reflexology has been enormously successful in providing relief for all muscular and skeletal conditions. It can provide pain relief, improve mobility, reduce inflammation and dispel toxins from the system. Sufferers find that they can often reduce their analgesics with regular reflexology.

It is interesting that stiffness in the foot represents stiffness in the body. As the feet are massaged so the muscles relax and the joints become more mobile.

ARTHRITIS

Osteoarthritis is the result of wear and tear of the joints and affects all of us to some extent particularly in later life.

Causes

* getting older!
* trauma to joints

Other advice

* keep joints mobile with regular gentle exercise such as yoga or Tai Chi
* eat a healthy diet as highly processed foods can lead to a build-up of toxic waste

Reflexology Treatment

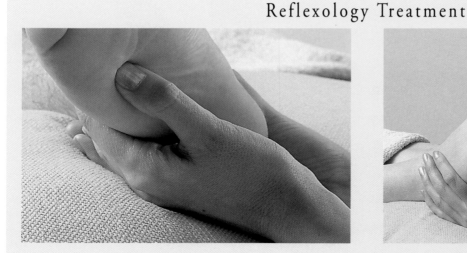

Solar Plexus

Adrenals

The whole foot should be worked as it is a general body condition. The following reflex points, however, should be emphasised.

* Kidneys – to eliminate waste materials that accumulate around joints
* Adrenals – to fight inflammation and give pain relief
* Solar plexus – to release tension (plus any joints which are affected)

GENERAL ACHES AND PAINS

Where there are problems with the muscles and joints the painful
areas should be treated as described below.

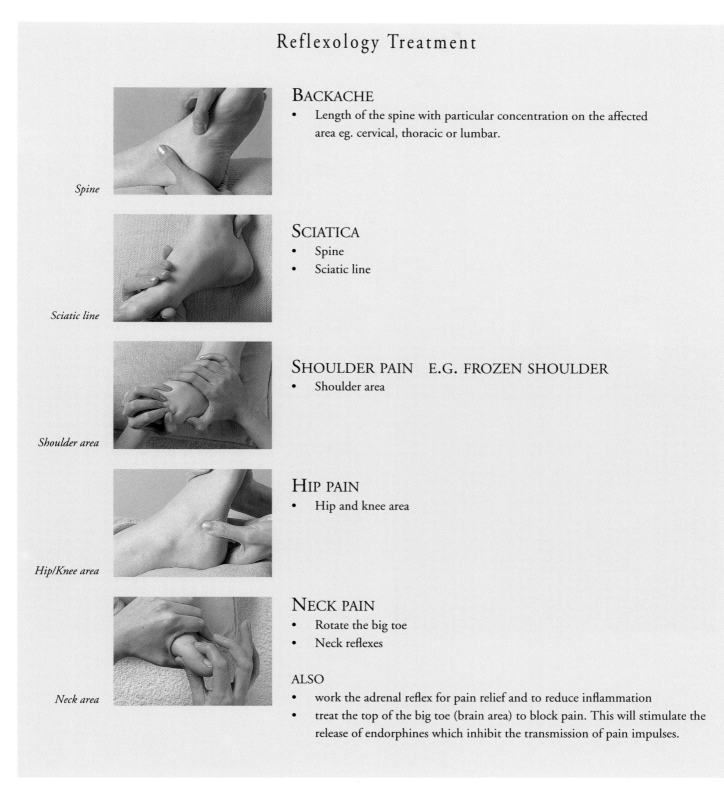

Reflexology Treatment

BACKACHE

- Length of the spine with particular concentration on the affected
  area eg. cervical, thoracic or lumbar.

Spine

SCIATICA

- Spine
- Sciatic line

Sciatic line

SHOULDER PAIN E.G. FROZEN SHOULDER

- Shoulder area

Shoulder area

HIP PAIN

- Hip and knee area

Hip/Knee area

NECK PAIN

- Rotate the big toe
- Neck reflexes

ALSO
- work the adrenal reflex for pain relief and to reduce inflammation
- treat the top of the big toe (brain area) to block pain. This will stimulate the
  release of endorphines which inhibit the transmission of pain impulses.

Neck area

RESPIRATORY PROBLEMS

All respiratory problems including simple coughs and colds, asthma, bronchitis, emphysema and other chronic bronchial conditions respond well to the regular use of reflexology.

ASTHMA

Asthma is becoming more prevalent particularly amongst children. It is characterised by wheezing and is due to inflammation of air passages in the lungs, causing narrowing of the airways and reducing airflow in and out of the lungs.

Causes
* allergies such as pollen, house dust, fur, feathers, certain foods or pollutants
* stress and anxiety may precipitate an attack

Other advice
* avoid dairy foods which increase mucus production
* breathing exercises should be practised daily. Most asthmatics breathe primarily from the chest while the lower portion of the lungs, which should be supplying 80% of the oxygen, is not used. Either sit up or lie down with one hand on your abdomen and one hand on your chest. Breathe in for approximately 6 counts and feel your abdomen fill with air and finally your chest. Hold the breath for two and then breathe out for 6 counts. The hand on the abdomen will move before the hand on the chest if you are performing this exercise properly

Reflexology Treatment

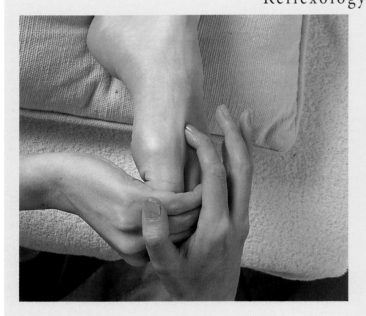

Lung/chest area

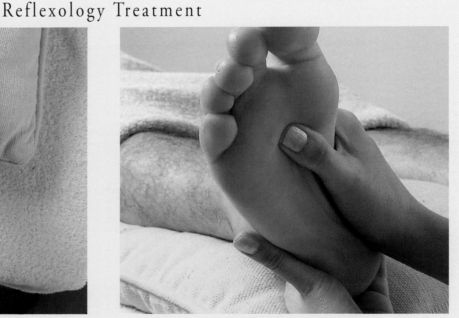

Solar plexus/diaphragm

* Lung/chest area
* Solar plexus/diaphragm – to release tension
* Adrenal glands – for allergies

COUGHS/COLDS/RESPIRATORY INFECTIONS

All of us will occasionally get a cold and reflexology is an excellent way of relieving the many symptoms and aiding the removal of mucus to prevent the occurrence of more serious conditions.

Causes

- exposure to viruses – schoolchildren have more coughs and colds due to exposure to lots of different germs and close proximity to each other

Other advice

- eat garlic which is known as 'nature's antibiotic'
- hot spices such as ginger will help to break down phlegm
- take vitamin C daily – at least 1 gram to prevent coughs and colds

Reflexology Treatment

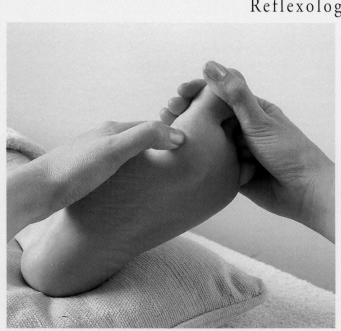

Thymus

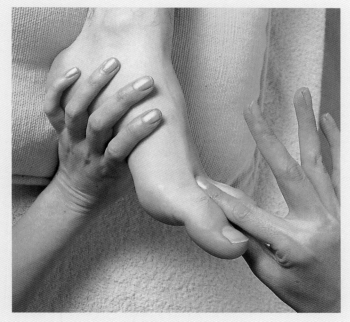

Lymph drainage

- Lung/chest area – to break up congestion
- Nose
- Throat
- Eyes
- Ears
- Thymus – to boost the immune system
- Lymph drainage – especially upper lymphatics

SKIN PROBLEMS

Skin disorders include acne, eczema, dermatitis and psoriasis and reflexology can help any skin condition. It improves circulation and so the skin should take on a healthy glow.

Causes
- hormonal imbalances
- dietary factors
- stress

Other advice
- avoid sugar, fatty foods and caffeine
- eat plenty of fruit and vegetables
- drink 6 - 8 glasses of water daily
- avoid stress
- never wear man-made fibres such as nylon next to the skin

Reflexology Treatment

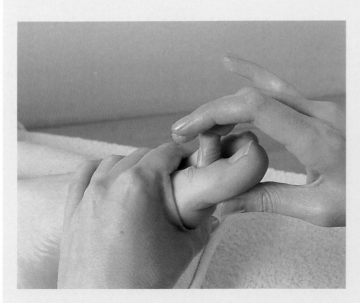

Face

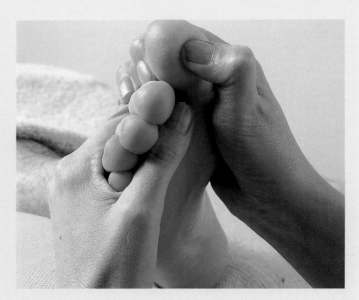

Pituitary gland

A complete treatment is beneficial to stimulate elimination of toxins but special attention should be given to the following areas:-

- Reflex zones relating to the area affected e.g. face
- Pituitary gland – to regulate hormonal activity
- Kidneys – to improve elimination
- Adrenal glands – to counteract inflammation
- Lymphatics – to cleanse the body

self Reflexology

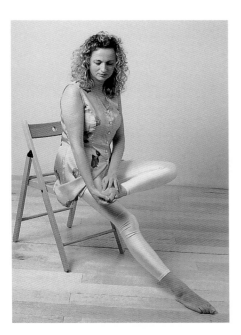

W hilst self-treatment is possible, it is virtually impossible to give yourself a complete treatment of foot reflexology. It is difficult to be able to relax sufficiently to derive the maximum benefit from a treatment. It is also very awkward to reach some of the reflex points.

When carrying out self administration there is not the exchange of energy which exists when one individual works on another. Therefore, it is much more relaxing and therapeutic to entrust your feet to the hands of another. However it is possible to treat a limited number of specific reflexes to relieve ailments such as headaches. So self-treatment can be very useful to achieve quick relief from a condition.

When you do work on your own feet sit down as comfortably as possible and surround yourself with pillows and cushions.

You need to be able to sit cross legged or at least be able to raise one foot on to the opposite knee so that you can see what you are treating. You may either sit on the floor, bed or on a chair.

The sequence below is excellent for de-stressing yourself and for general health care. It should take about ten minutes and can be done whenever you feel like it.

STEP 1   EFFLEURAGE THE FOOT TO RELAX AND CALM

Using both hands, stroke the foot, working upward from the toes towards the ankle bones (1) and back again (2).

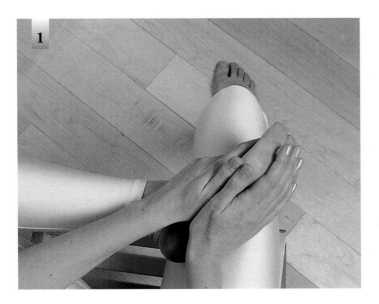

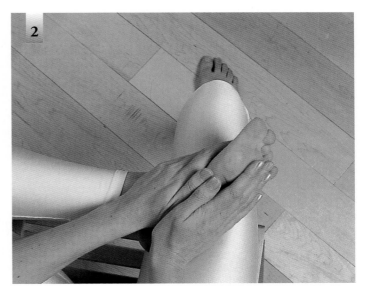

STEP 2 WALK THE SOLAR PLEXUS TO RELEASE STRESS AND TENSION

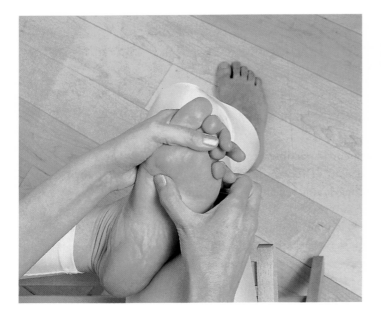

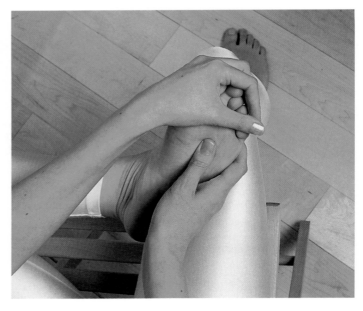

Wrap your fingers and thumb around the ball of the foot with your holding hand. Thumb walk across the diaphragm line.

When you reach the solar plexus press gently into it and gradually release the pressure.

STEP 3 THE SPINE

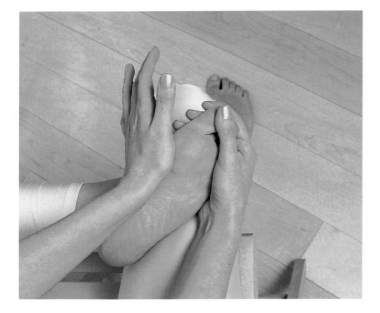

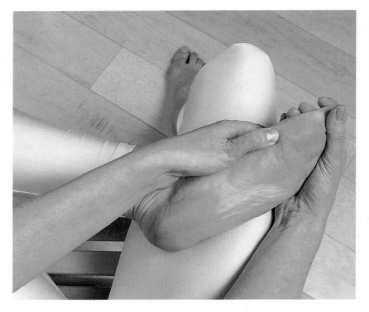

Stroke gently down the inside of the foot with the heel of your hand to encourage the spine to relax

Caterpillar walk up the inside of the foot working from the base of the heel up to the base of the big toe nail. You may walk in the other direction if you prefer. Pay particular attention to any areas which are sore.

STEP 4 NECK

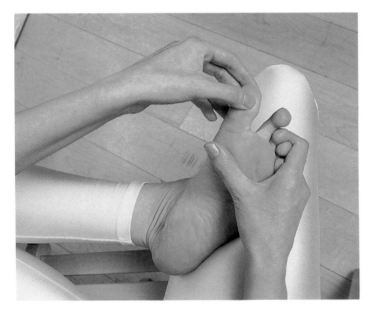

Hold the big toe between your index finger and thumb and gently rotate it clockwise and anti-clockwise to release tension and increase movement in the neck.

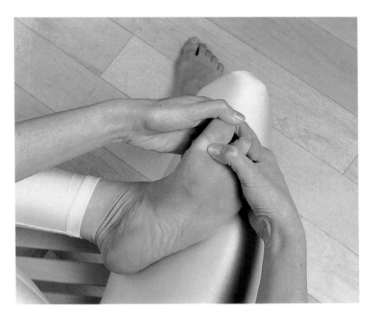

Thumb walk across the back of the base of the big toe and continue to walk across the front base of the big toe.

STEP 5 PITUITARY GLAND

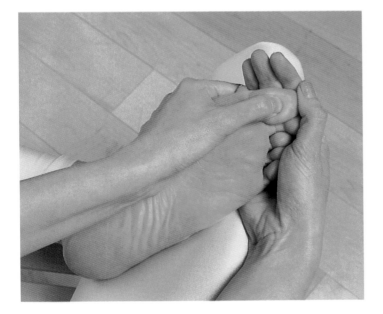

Locate the widest part of the big toe and the pituitary gland is found approximately at the mid-point of this line.

STEP 6 CHEST AND COLON BOOSTER

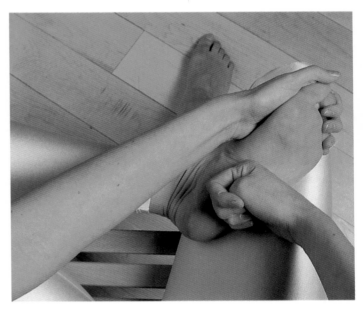

Make a fist with your hand and place it on the fleshy area on the ball of the foot. Use a gentle circular motion on the upper third of the foot to relax and decongest that chest area.

You may work on the lower third of the foot to encourage elimination of the colon. Excellent for constipation.

Step 7

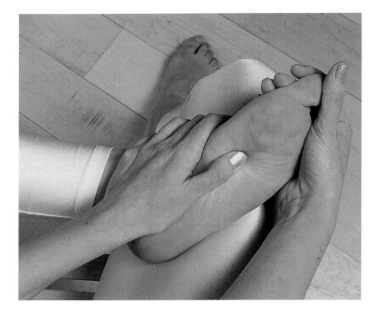

Treat any areas which need special attention. Here the kidney area is illustrated, but other common areas to come back to include the head and brain area if you have a headache and the stomach area if you have indigestion. Please refer to the relevant chapter for advice on treating specific ailments.

Step 8

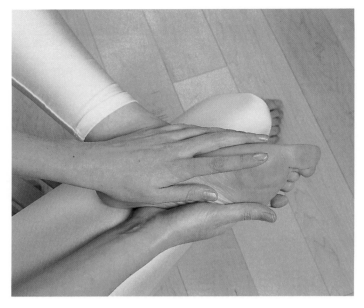

Effleurage the foot again to disperse any toxins which have been released.

Repeat the sequence on the other foot. Now allow yourself time to sit or lie back for at least 10 - 15 minutes.

Taking Care of Your Feet

Most us are fortunate enough to be born with a healthy pair of feet but by the time we reach old-age (and often before!) we have developed some kind of foot disorder. What is more it is probably self induced, perhaps caused by years of ill-fitting fashion shoes.

Feet are often the most neglected part of the body but now it is time to learn to take care of your feet. Not only will they look good but you will also feel much more healthy. If you bear in mind that every part of the foot represents a part of the body in miniature, you should look at any corns, calluses and athlete's foot in a new light. Is that athlete's foot between toes 2 and 3 affecting your eyes? Was that corn on the top of toe 4 there before or after you got that toothache? No wonder your neck has been playing up – look at the redness at the base of your big toe. So you should realise by now that you must be kind and considerate to your feet.

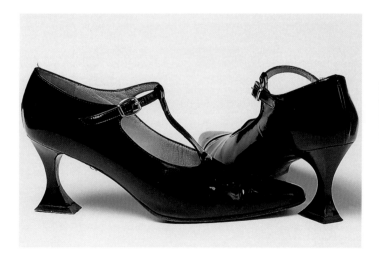

Fashion shoes are often responsible for foot disorders.

FOOT CARE TIPS

* Wash your feet daily to remove bacteria and dry thoroughly, particularly between the toes. This will help to prevent fungal conditions such as athletes foot from developing and also stops smelly feet. You may like to add pure essential oils to your footbaths. Add six drops of essential oil to a bowl of hand hot water just before you immerse the feet and soak for about 10 to 15 minutes.

Try the following recipes.

ATHLETES FOOT
3 drops lavender
3 drops myrrh

IMMUNE BOOSTER
3 drops lemon
3 drops tea tree

TIRED, SWOLLEN FEET:
3 drops chamomile
3 drops lavender

RESTORATIVE AFTER A LONG, HARD DAY
2 drops lavender
2 drops peppermint
2 drops rosemary

TO STIMULATE CIRCULATION
2 drops geranium
2 drops black pepper
2 drops mandarin

CRACKED OR CHAPPED FEET
3 drops benzoin
3 drops patchouli

COOLING
FOOT CREAM
To 30g cream add:

7 drops peppermint

CRACKED
FOOT CREAM
To 30g cream add:

3 drops benzoin
2 drops myrrh
2 drops patchouli

REMEMBER:

- Walk around barefoot as often as possible. Feet do not like to be confined in shoes all time. This will help to prevent foot deformities.

- Always cut your toenails straight across to stop ingrowing toenail from occurring.

- Use a pumice stone on the hardened areas to remove dead skin and prevent build up.

- Massage your feet and regularly with pure organic foot creams. You may use high quality pure essential oils for their healing properties. Try to avoid chemical foot sprays.

- Throw your shoes off at the weekend and walk on the grass or beach. This will make you feel grounded yet exhilarated.

- Avoid socks that are made of synthetic fibres such as nylon which make the feet perspire. Wear cotton and wool socks instead.

- Exercise your feet regularly to keep yourself supple and healthy.

TRY THESE SIMPLE EXERCISES EVERY DAY :

1. Rotate your feet in both directions to loosen them up and get rid of unwanted fluid around the ankles.

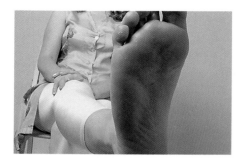 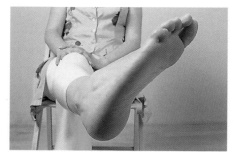

2. Walk on the balls of your feet especially if you have chest problems such as asthma.

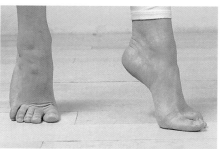

3. Pick up a pencil with your toes. This helps to tone up ligaments and tendons and also helps relax the neck and shoulder muscles.

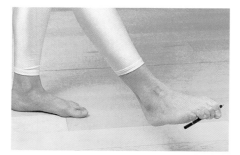

4. Place a ball under your foot and roll it the length of your foot. This will stimulate the respiratory and the digestive systems.

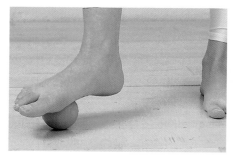 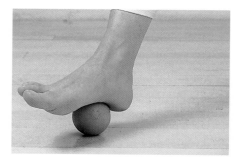

5. Walk on the outsides of your feet to keep them from rolling inwards.

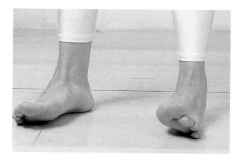

VISITING A REFLEXOLOGIST

Perhaps you would like to visit a professional reflexologist for a treatment. Check that your practitioner is fully qualified and insured rather than the product of a weekend workshop. Obviously the best way to choose a practitioner is by recommendation. Good practitioners are usually very busy so be prepared to wait a while.

The initial consultation can take up to one and a half hours. The reflexologist will take a detailed medical history and will also want to know about your lifestyle. Then your feet will be thoroughly examined for any imperfections which could indicate an imbalance of that reflex zone.

Then the treatment will begin and last approximately 30 to 45 minutes. At the end of the session you may be given self-help treatment to apply between sessions to achieve faster results.

All in all it should be a very pleasurable experience. Patients usually feel very light and euphoric and have a warm glow all over the body. What a wonderful relaxing way to restore optimum health!

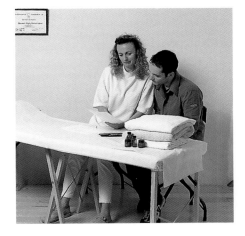

A reputable reflexologist will provide a detailed consultation before commencing treatments.

ADVANCED TRAINING

Once you have practised and mastered the techniques in this book, you should have been encouraged by the results you have achieved whilst working on yourself, your family and friends. Hopefully reflexology is now an integral part of your daily life.

If this book has inspired you then you may decide that perhaps you would like to become a professional reflexologist. The image of reflexology has dramatically changed over the last twenty years. When it first began to be known in the West during the 1980s it was regarded with a good deal of suspicion and scepticism. Nowadays the field of reflexology is accepted and well-known all over the world. Now students regularly include doctors, nurses, osteopaths, chiropractors, physiotherapists and psychologists as well as many lay people.

A recognised professional reflexology training will take at least nine months and will involve in-depth study in anatomy and physiology. The course should be accredited to a reputable reflexology association. Some schools simply issue their own certificates on completion of a course – these certificates can be worthless, expensive pieces of paper which are not recognised.

You should always check the qualifications of the principal. He/she should be a qualified teacher with AT LEAST five years clinical experience. Some individuals qualify and immediately set up their own courses without ever practising reflexology.
Never be afraid to ask questions if you are unsure about anything and perhaps arrange to go and see the College in action and look at the students work and case histories.

If you are unsure, it is always worth checking with the main reflexology institutes or organisations in your region or country.

PRIMARY REFLEXOLOGY ASSOCIATIONS

United Kingdom

Beaumont College of Natural Medicine
39-41 Hinton Road, Bournemouth, Dorset,
BH1 2EF, England
Tel: (44) 01202 708887

International Federation of Reflexologists
78 Edridge Road, Croydon, Surrey,
CR0 1EF, England
Tel: (44) 181 667 9458

United States

International Institute of Reflexology
PO Box 12642, St Petersburg, Florida, 33733-2642,
USA

Reflexology Association of America
4012 S Rainbow Boulevard, Box K585, Las Vegas,
Nevada 89103-2059, USA

CANADA

Reflexology Association of Canada (RAC)
Box 110, 541 Turnberry Street, Brussels, Ontario
N0G 1H0, Canada
Tel: (1) 519 887 9991 Fax: (1) 519 887 9792

AUSTRALIA

Reflexology Association of Australia
PO Box 366, Cammeray, NSW 2062, Australia
Tel: (61) 02 4721 4752

BOTH FEET

- tuning into the feet.

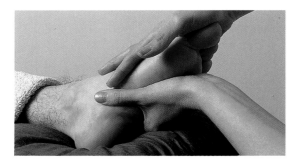

RIGHT FOOT

RELAXATION TECHNIQUES

- effleurage/stroking
- metatarsal kneading
- alternate thumb rotations
- zig/zag spreading the foot
- spinal stroking
- spinal twist
- toe loosening
- ankle rotations
- foot rocking

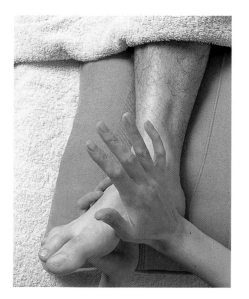

STEP BY STEP SEQUENCE

- solar plexus/diaphragm
- head and brain – thumb walk back and sides of the big toe
- pituitary gland – hook in and back-up technique on centre of big toe
- face – finger walk front of big toe
- neck
  - rotate big toe
  - thumb walk across back of base of big toe
  - thumb walk across front base of big toe
- sinuses – walk down the centre and two sides of the small toes
- teeth – finger walk down the fronts of the toes
- upper lymphatics – gently squeeze the webbing between each of the toes
- spine – caterpillar walk down the inside of the foot. Repeat walking up the foot
- eyes and ears – thumb walk along the ridge at the base of toes. Press into eye point – between toes 2 & 3, ear points between toes 4 & 5

SHOULDER GIRDLE TO DIAPHRAGM LINES

- thyroid, parathyroid, thymus – thumb walk ball of foot beneath big toe. Press thyroid point – centre of pad, parathyroid – over to the left slightly, thymus right of thyroid gland
- right lung/chest – thumb walk chest area from diaphragm line to shoulder girdle line on sole of foot
- right breast/lung/mammary glands – finger walk front of foot from base of the toes to diaphragm line

DIAPHRAGM LINE TO WAISTLINE

- liver/gallbladder – thumb walk triangular liver area between diaphragm line and waistline. Rotate onto gallbladder
- stomach/pancreas/duodenum – thumb walk from inside of foot to approximately the centre of the foot
- right adrenal gland – rotate onto adrenal gland

LEFT FOOT

BELOW THE WAISTLINE

- right kidney/ureter tube/bladder – circle over kidney point, turn thumb and caterpillar walk down towards inside of foot to bladder reflex
- small intestines – thumb walk from waistline to pelvic floor line.
- ileocaecal valve/ascending/ transverse colons – hook in and back-up on ileocaecal reflex, thumb walk up ascending colon, rotate on hepatic flexure, thumb walk across transverse colon
- right shoulder/arm/elbow/hand/ hip/ knee/leg – caterpillar walk up and down outer edge of the foot
- sciatic nerve line/pelvic area thumb walk down Achilles tendon area on inside of foot across hard heel pad and up Achilles tendon on outside of foot. Knuckle heel pad on sole of the foot
- uterus/prostate – pressure circles with index finger on reflex points between inner ankle bone and tip of heel
- fallopian tube/vasdeferens/lymph/ groin – thumb walk from inside of ankle, across the top of foot to outside of ankle and back again.
- right ovary/testicle – pressure circles with index finger reflex located midway between outer ankle bone and tip of heel
- effleurage/stroke right foot

RELAXATION TECHNIQUES

- effleurage/stroking
- metatarsal kneading
- alternate thumb rotation
- zig/zag spreading the foot
- spinal stroking
- spinal twist
- toe loosening
- ankle rotations
- foot rocking

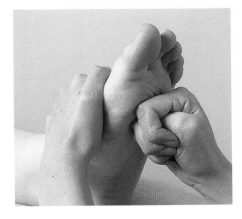

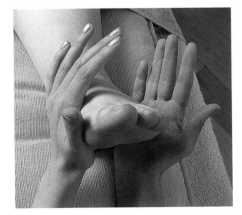

STEP BY STEP SEQUENCE

- solar plexus/diaphragm
- head and brain – thumb walk back and sides of big toe.
- pituitary gland – hook in and back-up on centre of big toe
- face – finger walk front of big toe
- neck
  - rotate big toe
  - thumb walk across back of base of big toe
  - thumb walk across front of base of big toe
- sinuses – walk down the centre and both sides of the small toes.
- teeth – finger walk down the fronts of the toes
- upper lymphatics – gently squeeze webbing between each of the toes.
- spine – caterpillar walk down the inside of the foot. Repeat walking up the foot
- eyes and ears – thumb walk across ridge at base of toes. Press into eye point between toe 2 & 3, ear point between toes 4 & 5

SHOULDER GIRDLE TO DIAPHRAGM LINES

- thyroid/parathyroid, thymus – thumb walk pad between big toe. Press thyroid point – centre of big toe, parathyroid over to the right slightly, thymus – left of thyroid gland
- left lung/chest – thumb walk chest area on sole of foot from diaphragm line to shoulder girdle line
- left lung/breast/mammary glands – finger walk front of foot from base of toes to diaphragm line
- heart area – thumb circles on upper third of sole of foot, index finger circles on top of foot

DIAPHRAGM LINE TO WAISTLINE

- stomach/pancreas/duodenum – thumb walk from the zone one to four from diaphragm line to waistline in horizontal rows
- spleen – thumb walk from a zone five to zone four in horizontal rows
- left adrenal gland – rotate onto adrenal gland

BELOW THE WAISTLINE

- left kidney/ureter tube/bladder – circle over kidney area, turn thumb and caterpillar walk to bladder area.
- small intestines – thumb walk in horizontal rows from waistline to pelvic floor line
- transverse colon/descending colon/sigmoid colon – thumb walk across transverse colon, walk down descending colon (zone five), just before pelvic floor line turn thumb to the left until you reach sciatic line, circle over sigmoid colon, caterpillar walk towards bladder area
- left shoulder/arm/elbow/hand/hip and/knee/leg – caterpillar walk up and down outer edge of foot
- sciatic nerve line/pelvic area – thumb walk down Achilles tendon on inside of foot, across hard heel pad and up Achilles tendon on outside of foot. Knuckle heel pad on the sole of foot
- uterus/prostate – pressure circles with index finger on reflex found midway between inner ankle bone and tip of heel
- fallopian tube/vas deferens/lymph/groin – thumb walk from inside of ankle, across the top of foot to outside of ankle and back again
- left ovary/testicle – pressure circles with index finger on reflex located midway between outer ankle bone and tip of heel
- effleurage – stroke left foot

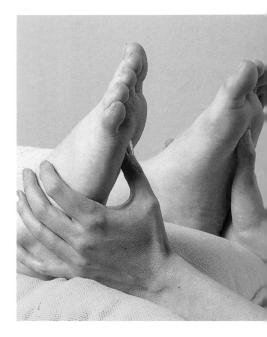

FINALE

- return to any reflex points which were tender
- perform any favourite relaxation techniques
- run fingertips lightly over both feet
- solar plexus release
- cover up feet and allow recipient to relax
- offer a glass of water and encourage recipient to drink plenty of water over next 24 hours

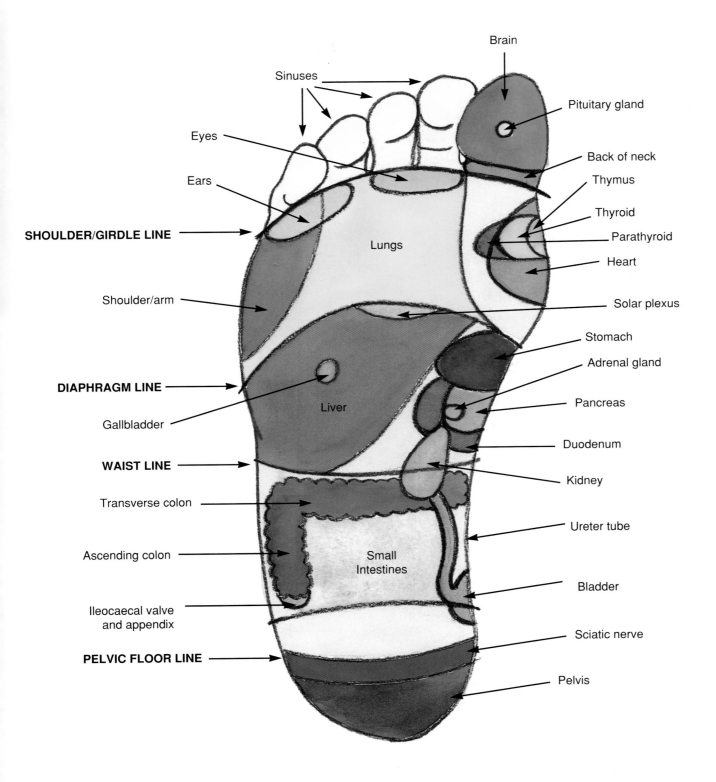

Brain

Sinuses

Pituitary gland

Eyes

Back of neck

Ears

Thymus

Thyroid

SHOULDER/GIRDLE LINE

Parathyroid

Lungs

Heart

Shoulder/arm

Solar plexus

Stomach

Adrenal gland

DIAPHRAGM LINE

Pancreas

Liver

Gallbladder

Duodenum

WAIST LINE

Kidney

Transverse colon

Ureter tube

Ascending colon

Small
Intestines

Ileocaecal valve
and appendix

Bladder

Sciatic nerve

PELVIC FLOOR LINE

Pelvis

RIGHT SOLE

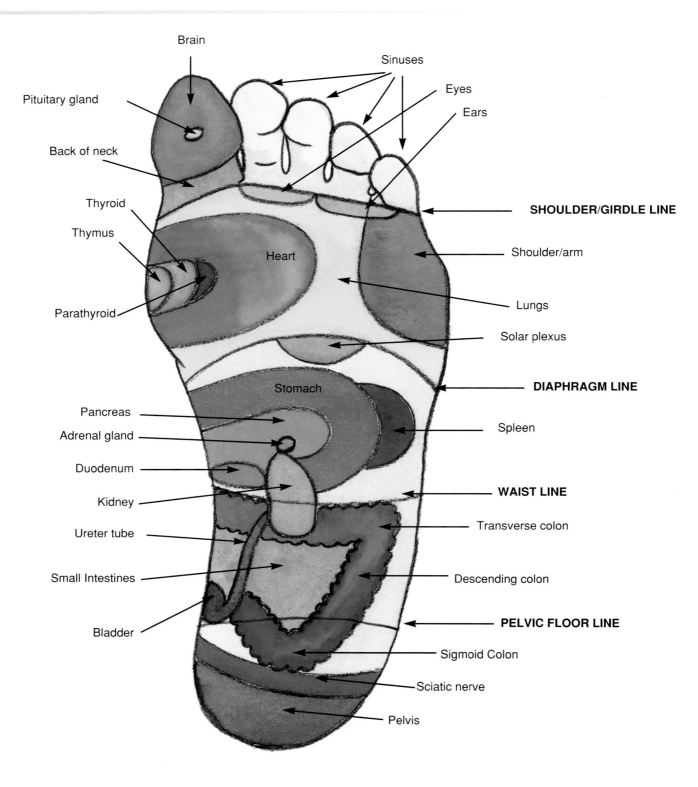

Brain

Sinuses

Eyes

Ears

Pituitary gland

Back of neck

Thyroid

Thymus

Heart

SHOULDER/GIRDLE LINE

Shoulder/arm

Parathyroid

Lungs

Solar plexus

DIAPHRAGM LINE

Stomach

Pancreas

Adrenal gland

Spleen

Duodenum

Kidney

WAIST LINE

Ureter tube

Transverse colon

Small Intestines

Descending colon

Bladder

PELVIC FLOOR LINE

Sigmoid Colon

Sciatic nerve

Pelvis

LEFT SOLE

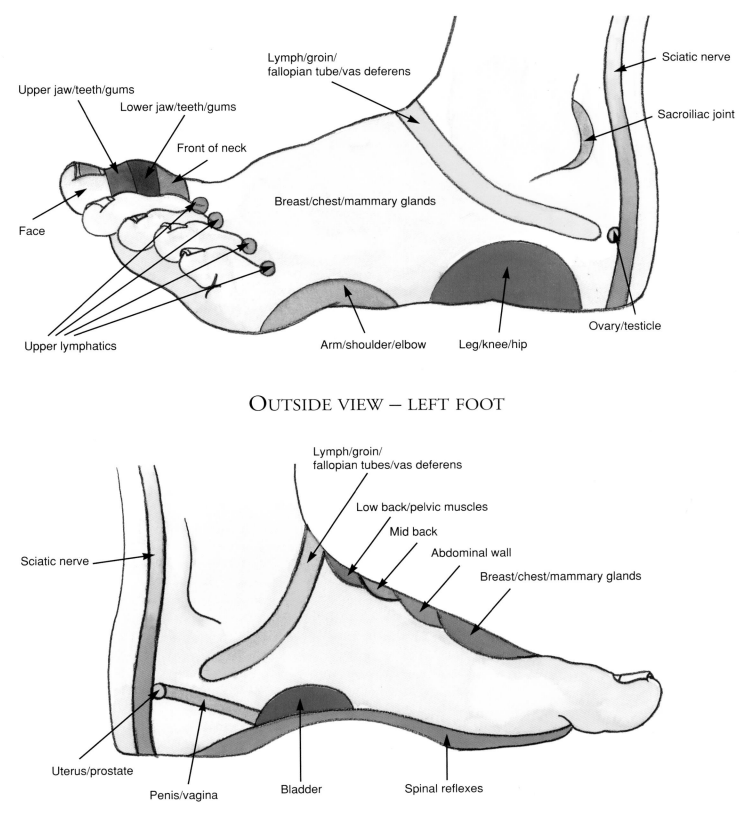

Sciatic nerve

Sacroiliac joint

Lymph/groin/
fallopian tube/vas deferens

Upper jaw/teeth/gums

Lower jaw/teeth/gums

Front of neck

Breast/chest/mammary glands

Face

Ovary/testicle

Upper lymphatics

Arm/shoulder/elbow

Leg/knee/hip

OUTSIDE VIEW – LEFT FOOT

Lymph/groin/
fallopian tubes/vas deferens

Low back/pelvic muscles

Mid back

Abdominal wall

Breast/chest/mammary glands

Sciatic nerve

Uterus/prostate

Penis/vagina

Bladder

Spinal reflexes

INSIDE VIEW – LEFT FOOT

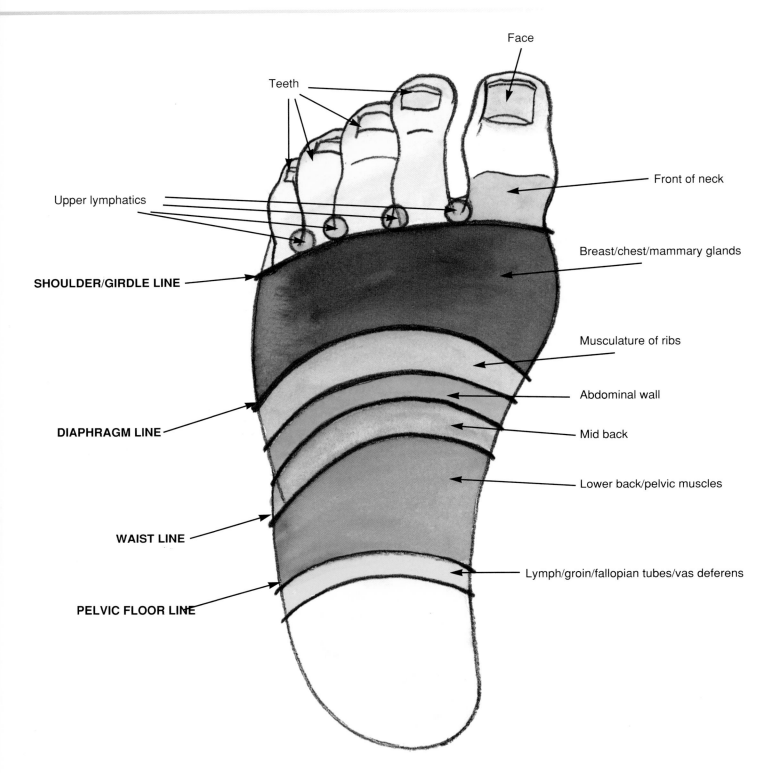

Face

Teeth

Front of neck

Upper lymphatics

SHOULDER/GIRDLE LINE

Breast/chest/mammary glands

Musculature of ribs

Abdominal wall

DIAPHRAGM LINE

Mid back

Lower back/pelvic muscles

WAIST LINE

Lymph/groin/fallopian tubes/vas deferens

PELVIC FLOOR LINE

DORSUM - LEFT FOOT

Index